Dear Royle—
Thanks so much for
your love & support over
the years!

Tales of an

Ugly Docling

#28

[signature]

Marie Duan Meservy

CONTENTS

A Dedication and a Humble Gift   i

Acknowledgements   vii

Foreword   ix

1   WHAT THEY DON'T TEACH IN MED SCHOOL

The Ugly Docling   2

Bedside Manners   5

Passage   7

Trauma, Death, and the Big Picture   9

Running With IV Poles   12

To Fight   14

2   ALONG THE CONVEYOR BELT AT THE DOCTOR FACTORY

The Secret to Success: Don't Buy Into "Talent"   20

I Will Never Eat Again   22

I'm Addicted to Studying   25

OB/GYN   29

How to Say Hello to a Crazy Person   33

I'm NOT an Alcoholic   36

How Surgery Is Like Psychiatry   40

Life After Getting Your Face Chopped Off   42

Pediatrics Chose Me   44

Stickers   45

Noah   46

My Hunger Diet   48

Death Is Optional! We'll Live Forever! So Far So Good!   52

A Bill From 3 Months Ago?   54

White Coat Syndrome   57

From Speed Dating to Wedding Day   60

A Honeymoon   65

Zigzagging   68

Medical School Is Not a Hobby   71

3 DOCTORS vs. PATIENTS

People Need Oil Changes Too   78

Life and Death   80

How to Win Friends and Influence Doctors   82

Delirium at 83   86

Holiday ER Stunt   89

4 ORIGINS AND DESTINATIONS

A Tiger's Parents   96

Roadmaps   99

Carpe Every Single Diem!   101

A Season For All Things   104

5 THE PROTAGONIST IS A RADIOLOGIST?!

An Explanation   110

How to Make Lifelong Choices: Don't Compare Apples and Oranges.   116
Just Make the Lemonade.

Pediatrics Personal Statement   119

Radiology Personal Statement   121

A DEDICATION AND A HUMBLE GIFT

Many people say that they're grateful to live in America, grateful to have freedoms and rights, schools, churches, big homes, fancy cars, and expensive hobbies. But most people have no concept of what it's actually like to be without these things.

When I was a little girl in China, I always dreamed of having a telephone in my own home. When my parents were first starting their careers as doctors, they had a tiny apartment with only one room, so I went to live with my grandparents in another city. I didn't get to talk to my parents at all except when they came to visit. (Telegrams were for emergencies only, and I didn't know how to read anyway.) When my parents moved into a slightly bigger place—an apartment in a dorm with a bedroom, a living room, and a small kitchen across the hall—I was finally able to move in with them. As a welcoming present, they took me to the mall and bought me my own toy telephone. I remember feeling like a princess! I would get together with neighbor children who also had toy phones and we would pretend to call each other; we have lots of pictures of me laughing on my phone. Years later, our neighbors next door installed a home phone; they were the first in our complex to do so. They could afford it because they were really important people. My dad moved to Canada around that time to get his Ph.D., and my mom and I had to stay in China while we waited for our visas. Once a week, my dad would call the neighbor's house to talk to us, and I felt lucky to be living so close to a phone. I would chat and sing him songs that I learned at school, and he would rack up an astronomical phone bill at the end of the month. Sometimes our neighbors would go out on the weekends, and my mom and I would know that we were going to miss dad's call. Those days it was sad every time we heard their phone ring. Years later, I moved in with my parents again, this time into a luxurious two-bedroom apartment in Montreal, and I had my own real telephone in my own room. Years later, my sisters and I signed a family cell phone plan with unlimited texting, because calling each other just wasn't good enough for them.

It's very humbling for me to think back on how I used to live, and even more so to imagine how my parents and grandparents used to live. I remember not having running hot water. I remember not having a refrigerator, and having to shop for just enough groceries for each day. I remember sharing a bathroom with several other families. I remember scrubbing my clothes on a washboard; I recently received a free washer and dryer because my friends thought it was a nuisance to have them sitting in their garage. It's wonderful how fast we can adapt to new improvements in our quality of life, and how many of those improvements bombard us all the time. And in some ways, it's wonderful that in America, we really don't see poverty. Right now, I may think being poor is having only $12 of "free spending" in my budget when I desperately want sushi for dinner. I don't think of those who make $12 in a whole month, or if I do, it is irrelevant because I don't even comprehend the meaning of living on so little.

Ironically, when I was little, my parents would tell me how fortunate I was to be born into good circumstances. I knew it, because when we went out, we saw the poor people in the streets; they were dirty, some were disabled, and all they owned was a bowl with which they would beg for food or change. And as far back as I can remember, I know my parents have always been extremely generous to others, sometimes unreasonably generous. I used to wonder why they were so nice, why they worked so hard just to let other people take advantage of them. I don't know the reason, but I think it's because after the poverty they have experienced growing up, they seem to remember that they own much more than a single bowl.

I think remembering this is key. Unfortunately, I know many individuals who call themselves poor, but I know very few people who aren't at least in the middle class. I certainly don't know anyone who lives on the streets. So it is truly a tragedy that *anyone* I know should call themselves poor at all! When we focus on ourselves and how we don't have enough, it's almost impossible to use what we do have to help others. Furthermore, I know that with such prideful ingratitude, it is impossible to be rich, no matter how much we have.

I look at my own life and I can't help but know that I am blessed. I have a great husband who cooks amazing dinners everyday. I have a supportive family. Aspiring medical students keep telling me I am lucky to be able to pursue my dream, and I feel fortunate to have the knowledge that I chose a career where I'm doing exactly what I should be doing in my life. And we may not have the latest smart phones or cable, but because we always live within our budget, we never, ever worry about running out of money—and so we never feel deprived. I try to remember the times when I was required to live with less, and when I remember, I am overwhelmed with how much I really have.

And of course I must remember the people who *do* have to live with less—much less—right now. **For so many, true poverty is not a memory but a reality. It is to these people that I dedicate this book.**

Because I am so grateful to have sufficient for my own needs, and because I feel it has been such a luxury to have the time and opportunity to write about my experiences as a medical student, I want to make my talent even more meaningful by making it a donation to the lives that need improving.

All of the proceeds of this work will be donated to medical charities, both locally and globally. If you've received this book as a gift, please consider making a small contribution to a medical organization. For a list of organizations that I support, visit www.uglydocling.com.

I hope that my messages, and any funds they generate, will reach many people in need. I also hope to never pay myself a penny for the time I've spent writing—that time has already been so rewarding.

ACKNOWLEDGEMENTS

Thank you, toaster! And blender, and oven, and dishwasher, and all other manner of labor-saving devices—THANK YOU! Without you, my medical career would not be possible.

Thirty years ago, as I gather from reading a female doctor's blog from the 1980s, medicine was a full-time occupation for two: a doctor and his housewife. The lady docs who tried raising children during medical school were made painfully aware of how they were doing it all wrong.

A hundred years ago, according to Wikipedia, it literally took all of a woman's time to housekeep. Think of putting a stick of butter on the dinner table: This would require milking a cow and churning by hand for hours while trying to keep it cold. And then they still had to bake the bread!

Today, females outnumber males in medical school. I can easily cook and clean while studying, and even write a book in my *real* spare time!

FOREWORD

I wondered for a whole year what I was going to title my book, and suddenly, "The Ugly Docling" came to mind. I think it's fitting on many levels.

For one, the Ugly Duckling is the story of a nerd kid who grows up to be a doctor (or engineer, or astronaut, or member of any profession that draws from the smart kid pool.)

I've been a misfit since elementary school. First it was because I was an immigrant, had an odd name, wore different clothes, and didn't speak the language. But even after I grew accustomed to American culture, I still struggled with being a nerd. I tried so often to dumb myself down so I could be accepted by other kids. I wanted people to know that I was a musician, a poet, and a tennis player, but I would be mortified if anyone found out that I was in MathCounts or Academic Olympics. And though I spent way too much time trying, I never had nice hair. For me, this one was tough; high school is all about the hair.

Fast forward to medical school: Everybody is a smartypants. Everybody is charismatic. Everybody has nice hair. Well, almost. When we tell people that we are going to be doctors, they react with kind words of admiration, appreciation, and respect. (And then they show us skin lesions for diagnosis.) Yet, when I found my old MathCounts roster and pointed out that a couple of my classmates were on it, they were mortified. It really is bittersweet to look back on those years. But hey, let's face it: Doctors don't just pop out of thin air; they were Mathletes when they were little! Nobody makes fun of a doctor. So why are American kids taught to make fun of nerds? I consider this book to be a big hug for my young self— and for nerd kids everywhere. **Nerd kids: It gets better!**

But my personal Ugly Duckling story continued even after I met up with the other swans in medical school.

Perhaps because of our common unspoken background as nerds, the culture in medical school is reversed. We admire and compliment each other for knowing the right answer at the right time. We fear being laughed at when we act ignorant or incompetent. Some may brag about how they never study, but they are either lying or willfully endangering lives and mocking the practice of medicine, and the rest of us know in our hearts that we would *never* refer our own patients to those individuals.

It was in this culture that I realized I may still be a misfit. Yes, of course I have studied my tail off, and of course I want other students to think of me as being a stellar student. But to the degree that I still have gaps in my knowledge, I question my doctoring skills. When I get an answer wrong, I question if all my classmates are smarter than me, if I can be a good doctor, if other doctors will want to refer their patients to me. For the first couple of years, I focused so much on test scores as measures of my doctoring skills. But then, when the exams were over and I was thrown into the real world of hospitals and clinics, I was humbled to learn so many things that were never taught in the medical classroom. *These* are the things that I felt moved to write about.

DISCLAIMER

The stories in this book are based on real clinical experiences, but in order to protect patient identity, all names, dates, and details have been changed.

1

WHAT THEY DON'T TEACH IN MED SCHOOL

Medical school proclaims to train doctors, yet the most valuable lessons and the greatest challenges pertinent to my career were never presented to me in classrooms or textbooks. I give these experiences the first pages of my book because of their importance in the kind of doctor that I have become.

The Ugly "Docling"

One time, an old Chinese gentleman was admitted to the ICU after being struck by a car. He was disoriented. He was deteriorating. He mumbled all kinds of crazy nonsense and wouldn't obey verbal commands. He seemed to get wilder every day of his hospital stay, so everyone thought his prognosis was very poor. When I started that rotation and was assigned to his care, I was really intimidated by his behavior. After reading in his chart that he was Mandarin-speaking only, I was even more intimidated, but I knew what I had to do.

The problem is, I have shied away from speaking Chinese in public ever since I moved to North America, so I still just have an eight-year-old vocab. (As a little girl, I was embarrassed to be Chinese. I learned English as fast as possible; I adopted an English name; I told people I was from Canada.)

Nevertheless, I did the best I could to act confident, addressing the patient by his Chinese name, pointing and using simple commands like "Can you lift this arm? What about this leg?" To my surprise, he listened and did everything I asked of him. That morning his Glasgow Coma Scale (a measurement of how well a trauma patient is doing) improved by 40% from the previous day—just by clearing the language barrier.

As I continued following his progress, he showed vast improvements. He was friendly, thankful, cooperative. He got out of bed for the first time in weeks and started functioning more like his old self. He even cleared the pneumonia he'd been fighting. Granted, he was still confused for a while, thinking he was in China. (Who could blame him? You'd probably think you were in China too if a Chinese medical student came to check on you every morning and spoke to you in Mandarin.) In the end, the doctors stopped expecting him to die in the hospital or a nursing home, and actually deemed him well enough to send home. The day he was discharged, he left us a big bag of chocolates and goodies (this was an exciting first for me.)

My superiors kept complimenting me for my management of this patient. Later I read on my evaluations, "Marie really bent over backwards for the team." But the funny thing is, I didn't! And I didn't feel it was any reflection of my "health care" skills, either! The patient healed on his own, I just helped motivate him by understanding him. The doctors managed the process, I just helped them better attend to his needs. I didn't study for this; I didn't plan for it in any way. I simply happened to bring something to the table that no one else could.

Is it any coincidence that what I had to contribute was what made me different as a little kid, the same thing that other kids used to tease me about? For once I can see how the Ugly Duckling feels when he grows up to be a swan, or how proudly Rudolph the Red-Nosed Reindeer comes to see his little red nose.

I guess that's the nature of having a red nose. Until we find a use for it, it just gets in the way. But without it, we really wouldn't be indispensable at what we do. And even for the ugliest of ducklings, a heritage can be as much of an asset as it had been a burden.

Bedside Manners

A motorcyclist crashed into a pole, and in the ER, it became my job to close the big laceration across his back.

Over the next half hour, I came to the room several times, irrigating and removing bits of rocks and debris, sewing stitches, and dressing the wound. After I'd asked all the usual questions (How did it happen? When was your last tetanus shot? Do you have any allergies?) we still had a lot of extra time.

So I just mentioned the next thing on my mind. "My brother-in-law rides a motorcycle also. We worry about him a lot." We went on to chat about family, and the places he'd been on his motorcycle, and what I did before med school. The EMT joined the conversation too.

I finished my stitches and said, "Thanks for letting me practice!"

As I walked away, I heard the EMT say to the patient, "That's the best kind of student to have practicing on you."

The patient replied, "Yeah, she was great! She did a really good job."

I thought that was pretty funny. Those sutures were on the patient's back. He never saw them, and he didn't have any way to know whether I had done a good job or not.

When I reported back to the ER doctor I was working with, he jokingly commented, "Well, looks like you won't be getting sued by that patient."

He was being sarcastic, but the point is a valid one. It is well known that patients judge the quality of their health care based on their relationships with their doctors. When it comes to lawsuits, patient unhappiness is a better predictor than poor health care. And so, making small talk is a vital component of sewing stitches.

In the ER, we talked a lot about malpractice and customer service. It was a touchy subject at times, because ER doctors perceived themselves as getting sued disproportionately more than their primary care colleagues. It seemed that in the face of a bad outcome, even if the primary care physician's negligence had resulted in the problem that was later discovered in the ER, a disgruntled patient more often sues the ER physician. The primary care physician has had years to build a rapport, and it's much easier to blame a stranger.

That's often how it goes in a doctor-patient relationship, though: One person holds the power of medical knowledge, but the other holds a much greater power of opinion.

Passage

A husband and wife were about to bring their first baby into the world. She lay across the surgery table. He sat with scrubs, cap and mask, anxiously waiting by her side. She grinned, even as her eyes glistened with tears. He spoke reassuringly as he squeezed her arm.

They had imagined this day over and over. Within minutes, with this birth, their lives would change forever.

A curtain of sterile draping fell between her head and abdomen, separating the excited parents from the hectic operation about to take place on the other side.

It was my first day in the OR since Anatomy dissections. She looked strikingly like a cadaver, except that she actually bled—multiple suction tubes flooded with blood. The OB with a flock of residents were frantically cutting, digging, and cauterizing.

"This is the uterus," they held up something huge and nodded at me. When they pierced it, amniotic fluid gushed out as if a hose had exploded.

From the chaos they pulled out a small bundle. The nurses rushed to it with a suction bulb and sucked the fluid from its mouth. Then it began to cry.

The dad stood up when he heard the sound. First his head emerged above the curtain, and then a video camera pointed in our direction.

I gasped. Everyone froze. Without missing a beat, the doctor held up the baby, smiling at the camera. Nurses quickly wiped off the blood. Then they swept the baby off to a table along the side of the room, and the video camera followed.

Work on the mother resumed. Placenta out, uterus closed, skin stapled.

The whole thing only took about twenty minutes. Nothing went wrong. It was a great case for a first-time medical student. And I found it to be horrific.

Only a thin veil separated the family's experience from ours. For them, a beautiful beginning of a new life together. For us, cutting and sewing and blood and guts. I almost felt it was out of place to say congratulations.

This is how I was born into the world of Medicine. I was thrown in headfirst, unprepared and alone. I would learn, over the years, that some of life's most precious experiences—birth, healing, death—are gruesome. I would witness many more than my share of such moments, again and again, as part of the routine of my career. I would struggle to find the beauty in the madness of this reality. Yet I would find it.

Trauma, Death, and the Big Picture

In the quiet hours of overnight call, I read this eulogy of Steve Jobs written by his sister. I was tickled to learn that on his ICU bed, Steve was inventing hospital gadgets:

"One time when Steve had contracted a tenacious pneumonia his doctor forbid everything — even ice. We were in a standard I.C.U. unit. Steve, who generally disliked cutting in line or dropping his own name, confessed that this once, he'd like to be treated a little specially.

"I told him: Steve, this is special treatment.

"He leaned over to me, and said: 'I want it to be a little more special.'

"Intubated, when he couldn't talk, he asked for a notepad. He sketched devices to hold an iPad in a hospital bed. He designed new fluid monitors and x-ray equipment. He redrew that not-quite-special-enough hospital unit.

"For the really big, big things, you have to trust me, he wrote on his sketchpad. He looked up. You have to.

"By that, he meant that we should disobey the doctors and give him a piece of ice."

Throughout my 31-hour shifts in the Trauma ICU, I marveled at how his sketch of Steve was just like the patients

I'd met: can't eat, can't breathe, can't move, but would like to go back to skydiving ASAP.

I think there are generally two types of ICU patients. There are the "vegetables" subsisting on life support, and the rest are feisty. The bull-rider with multiple spine fractures insists on bull-riding again the next day, even as he struggles to sit up. The teenager, whose ATV accident required brain surgery, asks me every hour whether we can take out the tube draining the bleed within his skull: "Will it be later today? Not 'til tomorrow? I can't sleep with this thing coming out the back of my head!" A man, whose brain is exposed by gaping holes in his head, tries to pull out every IV and monitor and walk right out of the hospital.

It seems as though these patients have an entirely different set of priorities than their doctors have for them. We want to manage their fluids and electrolytes. We want to make sure they have an airway. We want to save them from dying of pneumonia, of ischemic bowel, of cardiac arrest. But all they want is to continue whatever they were doing that landed them in the hospital in the first place. Don't they learn from their mistakes, and don't they realize that they can't live without these devices and measures we are taking for them?

But as damaging as it can be to a doctor's ego, I get it. I don't believe our work is more important than the lives we save. We bring out the defibrillators and ventilators to make people continue living, but that is not what I consider "saving a life." People don't live to have normal potassium levels measured in their blood. People live to bull-ride, to dirt bike, to invent computers, to be home with their families.

Obviously the basic needs have to be met in the hospital. It can be a cruel process, and patients may not get that ice cube after they've already starved for days, but we take great consideration in the treatment plan and believe that what we're doing is for the best. But after the healing is done, when bodily functions return to baseline, *then* what? Our story ends with the hospital discharge.

But the hospital discharge is the beginning of a longer road to recovery and *life*. Lots of changes and arrangements have to be made at home. The patient may be a burden to their family for a long time yet. That is why, beyond getting to leave the hospital bed, my hope is that these patients can survive to the next time they can do what brings them joy, whether it's strapping on a parachute or bouncing their child on their knee. To me, *that's* when their life has truly been saved, not a moment sooner.

Running With IV Poles

I wish I could show you a picture of this young couple huddled over the side of a crib. Their faces were clouded with deep concern. Their baby had spent the greater part of four or five years in various hospitals, for treatment of a multitude of problems. His endocrine problem, which brought us into the treatment team, was the least of these. Even though we were only monitoring one lab value, we came by to check on this little patient every day. Every single time, we walked into this same scene with his devoted parents huddled over his crib.

I wish I could show you a picture of this child. Like so many Pediatric Endocrine patients, he was tiny for his age. He lay floppy in his bed, barely able to move his claw-like limbs. And he had these fascinating buggy eyes that seemed to stare in opposite directions.

Parenting is complicated, of course. There are many tremendous tasks associated with caring for a child, and despite excellent efforts, children don't always turn out as one hopes or predicts. But, seriously, *no one* could have been prepared for this! And yet, I have never seen any parents who loved their kid more than these brave people loved this poor child.

Pediatrics can be a tragic, heartbreaking field to work in, especially at a tertiary care center like UCSF (where I was visiting at the time.) Every patient has several big problems. Too many will die shortly. Families have to split time between the hospital and the life they want. Parents put off their education, their careers, their relationships, their other children. They drag on in these horribly straining circumstances for months, years, indefinitely—until their trials end abruptly in the death of the little one. So many times a day I wonder how all these families make it through such times.

The beauty of Pediatrics is getting to be a part of these stories, to see example after example of courage and resilience, and to help bear these huge burdens in some small way. It's the little head poking around the IV pole, shouting, "Excuse me, Doctor, I can't see the TV!" It's the five-year-old grinning when asked about his new diabetes, then running over to bite his brother's head. It's the sigh and nod of a tired mother writing down the dosages of yet another new medication regimen. It's the gorgeous young couple huddling over the crib of their severely deformed son.

The beauty of Medicine in general is seeing people in the most unimaginably horrific circumstances, and realizing, they are just people. They are *not* a list of diagnoses. They are *not* limited in their ability to be happy.

To Fight

Have you ever had a doctor break down and cry with you as you received bad news? Sometimes I have to work really hard not to be that doctor.

On any given day in Oncology clinic, I might see all the stages of grief. Everyone battles cancer from a completely different angle, and I get to experience it all as one giant roller coaster.

One minute an old woman comes in after her last round of chemo left her hospitalized. She absolutely insists on taking another round. Her doctors hesitate to give her more chemo and radiation than she could tolerate, yet she refuses to go to the grave without having pulled out all the guns. The defiance in her eyes is contagious. I want to shout, "Yeah!! Go get 'em!"

Next thing we meet a young man whose cancer had no business interrupting the course of a well-plotted life. He's already nauseated just worrying over how the treatments will affect his family. He and his wife raise a slew of questions, exploring every crevice of every possibility. Our uncertainty makes them visibly uneasy: Curing cancer may be a numbers game from our perspective, but for each individual patient, we either achieve a cure or we do not. For this couple, the side effects are definitely not worth it for a not-cure. I wonder if he might talk himself out of getting any treatment at all.

Then we get a happily oblivious patient, a guy with brain tumors so far gone that he no longer has the capacity to understand his own plight. We try to explain that he needs to take his chemo pills diligently. He smiles pleasantly and agrees, from which we gather that he won't do anything of the sort. While this is truly terrifying to me, part of me also thinks that perhaps, for a cancer patient, he is in the best of all possible worlds.

The tearful patient really gets to me. Someone had given her false hopes about her prognosis, so then it became our job to set the record straight. The doctor apologizes profusely. The patient retreats into heaves and sobs as she begins to mourn her own death all over again. In her mind, we have just killed her. I hand her a box of tissues—inadequate for the gravity of the situation. Yet she smiles briefly as she takes the box from me. We continue the conversation as she empties the box. Pagers ring, and we silence them without answering. Occasionally I stare at the ceiling so the tears won't crash down.

A flurry of questions tear through my mind: Where in my medical training was I supposed to learn how to let a patient die? How do I tell the dark news, and then how do I react? Do I grieve the disease, or do I fight it? What does the patient need to hear? Is it inappropriate to laugh with them?

To cry? Is it unprofessional to admit that the cancer, in beating the patient, is also beating the doctors?

What is a good doctor?

2

ALONG THE CONVEYOR BELT AT THE DOCTOR FACTORY

This is an account of the adventures I've had during these four years from medical school orientation to graduation. Those who judged this book by its cover will likely find what they are looking for in this section.

The Secret to Success: Don't Buy Into "Talent"

Have you ever heard of Histology? On my first day of medical school, I hadn't. I sat through four hours of Histology lectures and two hours of Histology lab. I was overwhelmed. I couldn't type fast enough. I assumed I was the only one who had no idea what was going on. I went home and Googled "histology" before launching into a ten-hour study session. Thus my medical career began.

When the results of my national board exam came back two years later, Histology was one of my strongest areas. I wouldn't have guessed it in the beginning, because learning it was always such a struggle.

Almost everyone is smart in medical school, but not everyone does well. Some of the smartest people in my class had their first round of medical school applications wait-listed or even rejected, while some of the highest pre-med achievers could barely scrape by. What determines our success here? I believe it's how much we choose to dig in. The truth is, none of us were born knowing the things we are learning now. Our job is simple: Figure out how best to study, and then keep at it.

For me, this affirms the realization that there is no such thing as "talent" and "intelligence" anymore. Those things mattered in high school maybe, when things were easy enough we could cruise through just by being smart. But after we've reached a certain level of achievement, it's all about perseverance. It was an empowering realization to make, one that was critical to my success.

I think this applies in any domain. Inborn gifts can only take us so far (and honestly, without practice, that is not very far.) Conversely, we are never so limited by our lack of talent that we couldn't make up for it with hard work. If we view our setbacks as a greater opportunity for growth, there is no reason we couldn't exceed all expectations and come out even farther ahead. The sooner we figure this out, the more empowered we are to become what we dream of being.

I Will Never Eat Again

When my husband asked what I wanted for dinner, I stated firmly that we were not to have meat on Anatomy days. He kindly decided to cook up a "vegetable soup," but unfortunately didn't realize the significance of the ingredients "shrimp paste" and "fish sauce." I got one whiff and immediately gagged. Still, determined to be appreciative, I dipped my spoon into the bits of shrimp. I was promptly bombarded with images of human carcass swimming in preservative bath. Though I was starving, I decided that eating was not for me. Later, he made me a new dinner: breakfast.

I have often chuckled as I reflected on that first day in Anatomy lab as a first-year medical student. Everybody wanted to be so brave, and yet, everybody seemed so squeamish! What we sincerely wanted to portray was, "Yes, I'm going to be a doctor. I like blood and guts and cutting people open!" But the shaky hands, awkward conversations, and nervous laughter must have given us away.

From behind me, my dissection partner exclaimed, "I see dead people!" It was both amusing and horrifying.

Truth is, despite having been a mouse heart surgeon in my previous life, and despite having come to medical school for the very purpose of becoming a surgeon, I got a creepy feeling working with the cadavers.

Surgery is an acquired taste. Each day, I have to become newly accustomed to the look, the smell, of open flesh. I have to tell myself, "Calm down. We are cutting a person. And that's okay." But death is a taste I may never acquire. A dead person, to me, is not okay. And just as well: A living patient is a sign of a good doctor, is it not?

It was hard for me to sort out in my mind how we were supposed to be learning to heal people by cutting them apart. I was overcome by a strange sense of guilt, like I was hiding a violent crime. I kept dreaming about cadavers—cadavers talking, cadavers coming to life, cadavers feeling pain. I got freaked out when I would turn over in bed and unexpectedly run into my husband's arm, or even my own arm. It was maddening. I felt like the cadaver was dissecting me and stripping away my sanity.

There was also the feeling that we were intruding. These people had no privacy; they couldn't hide anything from us. We saw their lung cancer, their prosthetic hips, their breast implants. Perhaps they didn't know they only had one kidney. I'm sure they couldn't care less. They had already played out their lives and we were nothing to them but one last charity case. And yet, we were getting to know them better, in a way, than they, their spouses, and their mothers ever knew them.

For the sake of patient privacy, these donors were presented to us without names, without any identifying information except whatever we could infer from the state of their bodies. Yet it was obviously and undeniably personal to open someone up, to handle their organs, and to understand their identity in that direct way that they never could themselves.

Exam after exam after exam... Gradually we became casual in our dealings with the cadavers. No one cringed when the instructional dissection videos would be shown on the big screen during lunch. We considered which of our classmates were muscular enough to make good cadaver specimens. One of my friends also wanted to become a surgeon; we each claimed one side of the cadaver and had an ongoing contest to see which side was dissected better.

Personally, I knew I'd been transformed beyond repair when I would consistently alienate my husband at the dinner table by my incessant talk of Anatomy.

I'm Addicted to Studying

Seriously. I have thought about this, and I'm pretty sure I meet clinical criteria for addiction when it comes to studying.

Consider these criteria for "substance dependence" (and kindly think of studying as a substance for the purposes of this discussion.)

1. Tolerance, as defined by either of the following:
- An increased amount of the substance is required to achieve the same effect.
-A decreased effect results when the same amount is used.

I first tried studying when I was in elementary school. I liked how it made me feel. I got a buzz from being smart, like I was on top of the world, and often I could see things that other people couldn't. But as time went on, it took more and more studying to get that same feeling. Now I'm in medical school, studying 40, 60, 80 hours a week in order to feel smart. I can't just feel smart after studying for half an hour, like I did when I was young.

2. Withdrawal, as manifested by either of the following:
-The characteristic withdrawal syndrome occurs.
-The substance is used to relieve or avoid withdrawal symptoms.

When I don't study, things can get out of hand. I start to feel resentment toward the people (usually family members) who are taking up my time and keeping me from studying. I get anxious about what's left of my evening and when I will get to study again. I get headaches, sometimes I lose my temper. If it goes on for a long enough time, I can even get delirious and do things that are completely out of character—like shopping, baking, or scrapbooking.

3. The substance is used in increasingly larger amounts, or over a longer period of time, than desired.

Sometimes on a Friday night, I think, "I'm just going to study a little bit, since it's the weekend and I have plenty of time." Monday morning hits and I am left wondering how I managed—yet again—to get nothing done besides studying all weekend.

4. The patient attempts or desires to decrease use.

Believe me, I've tried many times to cut back on my studying habit. I've stayed clean for a couple weeks at a time, maybe even for a whole summer. But it's only a matter of time before I go back to the same old environment, with classrooms and teachers and all my friends who are studying... and I always cave in again.

5. A significant amount of time and resources are spent obtaining, using, or recovering from the substance.

I know that I have spent a lot of time, and even squandered my life's savings, on studying. Textbooks are at least $50-100 a pop "on the streets." Sometimes you can get them cheaper, but you don't know what's been put in them (scribble marks, highlighting.) And I don't have a job, so I can't keep up with how fast I go through them. I've ended up in a lot of debt!

6. Important social, occupational, or recreational activities are given up or reduced because of substance use.

I try hard to make time for family and other things. Sometimes it hurts their feelings when I don't make it to their golf games, or to their graduation dinner, or to their wedding. I can't seem to hold down a job for long either because I end up studying so much. And that's too bad. I really do mean well at heart.

7. The patient has knowledge that the substance use is detrimental to his health, but that knowledge does not deter continued use.

Sure, I know that my habit is going to kill me sooner or later. I don't always sleep, or eat, or use the restroom when I know I should. I keep studying even when I am sick. I just... can't help it.

OB/GYN

I had all these expectations for how life would be for a third-year medical student: strutting around the hospital in a white coat stuffed with books and snacks, answering obscure questions on morning rounds, assisting in heroic surgeries, saving lives day in and day out. Before I knew it, six weeks in Las Vegas had come and gone. The adventure had been exhilarating and exhausting, but nothing like I'd expected.

I started off with two weeks on the Gynecology service. The entire first week was a blur of navigation: constantly getting lost in the hospital, hunting down patient charts, deciphering doctors' handwriting, figuring out what information I needed to write a note, looking up abbreviations on my new Android phone, gauging social interactions with new residents and new attendings. Actually, there weren't that many patients to cover, but the shock and the reality were quite enough to deal with. There were days we stood in the OR for ten hours straight, going from surgery to surgery to surgery. I lost track of how many hysterectomies I saw. By the second week, I had the logistics down and could actually develop my clinical skills. I had always been comfortable talking to patients, but getting all the relevant information in a timely manner, without getting sidetracked or confused from all the extraneous information, without forgetting anything, all at 5 AM, was really a matter of art. *Valuable lesson: Patients are just people—listen to them like you would listen to a friend.*

The next two weeks were spent catching babies on the Labor and Delivery floor. First, I had an 84-hour workweek, during which I helped fourteen babies arrive in this world (seven vaginal deliveries and seven C-sections including two emergencies.) It was an amazingly smooth series of events from my perspective: I would pick up a patient in triage, she would get admitted, and several hours later she would have a baby. I started timing myself when seeing patients; I had my history and physical down to fifteen minutes, and my progress notes down to five minutes. The second week was a little slower, and I had to leave the floor for hours at a time to attend lectures and give presentations, so I actually missed out on four deliveries. But I got to do two full deliveries by myself from start to finish, including an episiotomy repair. My total baby count was nineteen (eleven vaginal and eight C-sections.) *Valuable lesson: Nurses are wonderful—be gracious and submissive to them, and your life can be amazing.*

The last two weeks were spent in clinics, managing pregnancies and women's health. Lots of pap smears, pelvic exams, ultrasounds. Lots of diabetes and hypertension. Also lots of studying in between patient visits. The highlight of my last week was seeing one of my surgery patients from a month prior. She was an elderly lady who came in anemic and looking pregnant, and was diagnosed with leiomyosarcoma—a cancer of the uterus that had spread to her ovaries, intestines, bladder, and stomach. She was devastated, but handled everything bravely. It was a long operation trying to take out as many of the tumors as possible, and she stayed in the hospital for several days afterwards. She got used to me waking her up at 5 AM to check on her, and despite being tired, weak, and in a lot of pain, she would diligently push herself up to sitting so I could listen to her lungs. When she returned to clinic for her six-week follow-up, she was energetic and happy. She wore a clean white dress and a flower in her hair—a drastic difference from the feeble grandma in a smelly hospital gown that I remembered. And she asked many concerned questions about how my education was going; she said she didn't know what she was signing up for when she agreed to let a medical student take care of her, but she was really glad she checked that box. *Valuable lesson: Be competent and confident, but above all else, be kind.*

Overall, a fascinating time of putting together different sets of knowledge and being kept on my toes. In the first two years of medical school, I had been taught more disease processes than I will ever see as a doctor. But in the first two clinical months I learned that the diseases were all connected by the thread of human suffering.

In my job, all efforts are mustered to relieve that suffering. This is what being a doctor is all about: combining the science of clinical skills and tools with the art of understanding people.

How to Say Hello to a Crazy Person

I routinely meet people at the most dramatic, pivotal moment of their lives: They have just had a brain malfunction that got them locked up in a hospital against their will. They want to go home, but in order to do so, they first have to prove to me that they are normal. The whole idea of having a psychiatrist talking to them can be unsettling, if not downright offensive. I must say I have never before had to be tactful, even apologetic, in the simple act of introducing myself. Unfortunately, it's not as easy as one might think. It goes something like this:

"Hello? Mr. ___?"

At least once, I have been greeted with a warm "Get out!" or, better yet, a clipboard chucked across the room. I then quickly assess my safety: Am I within striking distance? Does the patient have another hard object to throw at me? If I am safe, I muster my resolution to get that history, and continue:

"My name is Marie, and I am a medical student from the Psychiatry service. I'm just here to see how you're doing today. Did your primary care doctor tell you he has asked me to come talk to you?"

The answer to this question tells me a lot about someone's mental status. I have gotten everything from "Oh, good! I've been waiting for you!" to "You're not going to ask me to spell 'world' backwards, are you? I have Parkinson's, I'm not dyslexic." to "Are you a United States citizen? For how long? Can you prove it?" Depending on how I am received, I may have to backtrack and repeat this step several times, rephrasing, making jokes, offering reassurance, basically anything short of bribery to convince the patient that it's really in their best interest to talk to me. They are free to choose, but their treatment is halted, and, in many cases, they cannot legally leave the hospital, without clearance by Psychiatry.

If I get past all these security features and the patient agrees to an interview, I am in luck! I pull up a chair, making sure I sit between the patient and the door, and begin with an open-ended question:

"What brings you in today?"

And here, the patient will either tell me what is wrong: "I caught my girlfriend messing around on me and I tried to hurt myself," or will tell me something that lets me infer what is wrong: "My son brought me in when I was watching these nice people put on a Shakespeare play in my back yard." Sometimes the patient tells me nonsense that makes it clear something is very wrong: "I drank three shots of whiskey. I always do that before I go to work. Why did I black out? What am I doing here? Why am I covered in blood?"

I invite them to say more: "What made you feel so bad that you thought the only solution was to kill yourself? How did you react when you first noticed that your guts were rotting from the inside? Do you agree with your daughter that these voices aren't real, or are you not sure at this point?" Over the course of half an hour, an hour, sometimes longer, I find myself building an alliance with these people. Often the ones who were most adamant that I go away, turn out to be the chattiest.

The stories are enriched with sub-plots, sidetracks, opinions and obsessions, often clouded by poor insight, occasionally peppered with true psychotic symptoms like voices and visions. I have to piece it all together and, together with the team, decide whether and how we can make this person whole.

Within a week of working for the Psychiatry service, already my mind had been thoroughly provoked and my humanity thoroughly questioned and tested. Whether we would visit one or ten patients in a day, I took away dozens of stories that I yearned to tell.

I'm NOT an Alcoholic

I went to an Alcoholics Anonymous meeting. Not only that, but I also asked someone to be my sponsor. It was more or less a dare. I don't drink; I've never been a drinker in my life. I saw this as a fun social experiment, but I still couldn't help feeling out of my element. I sat down and introduced myself as a medical student—an observer. I'm NOT an alcoholic. AA is something I will prescribe to my alcoholic patients. I don't personally need to be here. I just had to come to fulfill an assignment.

Well, apparently that's how each alcoholic feels when they first come to AA. Our director on the Psychiatry rotation really believes in making us walk a hundred miles in the patient's shoes.

The meeting started off with everyone reading from the Big Book. As each person took their turn to read, they introduced themselves: "I'm Bob and I'm an alcoholic." Then the class replied, "Hi Bob!" Just like in the movies!

The chapter, which most of the members described as their least favorite, was an instructional letter to the employers of alcoholics. It talked about how to deal with people in your company who are draining the system by not showing up to work, being hungover, etc. First, you have to recognize that alcoholism is a disease, and you should think of your alcoholic just like you would think of your diabetic: Is this a good employee independent of his drinking problem? If not, fire him. Next, you should see if he is willing to quit. If not, fire him. But if he is worth keeping and he is willing to quit, you should take steps to ensure he gets medical and psychological treatment. Detox is relatively quick and easy, but then he will have to make a change of heart. You should talk to him afterwards, let him be honest about his wrongdoings and make restitution as appropriate. You should give him a fair chance to be better. Make it clear to him what your expectations are, and what the consequences will be if he messes up. But you should not adjust your standards for him and make him your "favorite." You just treat him like you would treat anyone else — with or without a disease. And if he slips after all this, then you can fire him and feel good about it!

I got the sense that alcoholics are just people. They should be regarded as such, no more, no less. I guess it's a hard transition for people to realize that, which is why a whole chapter was written in the Big Book about it. As one alcoholic said, "It's unrealistic to expect employers to read this book in the first place. Most of them say, 'You're an alcoholic? You're fired!' They don't want to go through all this."

I realized that it must be really hard for recovering alcoholics to assimilate back into society, even after they have made the commitment and necessary changes to rid themselves of the disease. I asked my sponsor, "Is it harder for you to be accepted again once you've labeled yourself an alcoholic? Do you find people making assumptions about you based on who you used to be?" To my surprise, he answered, "I don't mind being labeled an alcoholic by my boss and coworkers. I openly tell people that I am an AA member. My boss knows I've been through the process. I am a hard worker. I am the one who comes in at 6 AM. He has me talk to other employees about their habits. There is one guy who never knew about AA before, but is now actively involved in the program. I am happy that I can reach out to other people in this way and help them to overcome their addictions by sharing my own experiences. Sure, there are some people who are ignorant and have prejudices. I just make sure I don't bring it up to them again."

In this statement I gained a profound understanding of the entire essence of the 12-step program and of generally teaching others through example: Instead of viewing alcoholism as an imperfection that he has to hide, this man accepts his past as part of his identity. He uses his experience as an example to others. He teaches them the lessons he's learned, so they don't have to repeat his mistakes.

Everyone struggles with their own set of weaknesses. Some worship substances (aka "addiction,") some worship immorality (aka "sin,") some worship themselves (aka "pride.")

Many of us, through painful experience, learn to rise above those weaknesses. But why do we want to sink into anonymity with our shortcomings? Instead of covering up and pretending to have been perfect, how much better can we all become if we could be honest and humbly share how we were made stronger? As you can see, this AA observer has gained a valuable insight from an alcoholic. Time will tell how this will change me for the better.

How Surgery Is Like Psychiatry

My first week on the Surgery unit, a delirious patient began wandering the halls unattended, eventually creeping into another patient's room. Thinking he had found his wife, he then tried to crawl into bed with this other patient. Security was called, it was documented in the chart that the man was a danger to himself and others, and he was promptly moved to the Psychiatric floor where he was secluded in a locked room. Well, the other patient was a gentleman in his 80's, and severely demented, so he in fact did not seem to mind or realize what had happened.

Yes, I am indeed talking about the Surgery unit. Maybe crazy people are just everywhere. But more and more, I find there actually is a lot of common ground between Surgery and Psychiatry. For one, they both look inside people.

As I'd alluded to in my Anatomy reflections, seeing someone from the inside is both a privilege and a burden. When I'm armed with a scalpel, there is nothing that a person can choose to hide from me—I can see the entirety of the disease that ails them, I can assess the present, I can infer the past.

And now, from a surgeon's perspective, I can help to shape the future. Working with patients in the middle, rather than the end, of their lives is rewarding in many ways. We can help them, we can fix them, we can change how it ends for them.

I really revel in the gratification of bringing a patient to the operating room. They came to the hospital suffering tremendous pain. We did some tests and figured out the problem—something wrong with how they were built, or something that happened to mess them up. They were distraught when they found out. Some of them cried all the way to the OR. But then, we dug in. We looked inside, tweaked them, and removed the problem. And then they could function in the world again like they couldn't before.

You can imagine how I view Psychiatry as a similar process, prodding with words sharper than knives. The approaches may seem opposite. But in all of my experiences, the most sick, the most mangled patients of all have been Surgery and Psychiatry patients. And the two solutions are by far the most invasive in all of medicine.

Life After Getting Your Face Chopped Off

Yes, I too was shocked to learn, there *is* such a thing!

A guy came to our clinic with extensive oral cancer. He'd already had the mass removed once and undergone chemotherapy, but it came back. He was a relatively healthy young man, and quit smoking as soon as he was diagnosed. Initially he didn't want any surgery done, but he slowly changed his mind as he got sicker and ran out of options.

As he lay on the operating table, different teams of surgeons making plans and negotiating over his head, he looked scared. I went over and asked him, "Are you ready?"

He laughed. "Of course I am. Are *you* ready?" He had seen me reading in the pre-op room earlier and was quite pleased when I told him I was studying up on his case.

None of us knew that those would be his last words. But after six hours of careful dissection of the tumor and surrounding lymph nodes, the guy literally didn't have his tongue anymore.

When the operation was over, he couldn't articulate beyond grunts and vowel sounds. He wasn't able to swallow either, but instead would have to feed through a tube. I don't think anyone could have been ready for that.

When I saw him days later, he was still smiling. He'd stayed in the hospital over Thanksgiving weekend. Every day, nurses, students, and doctors had come by to check the pulse on his newly-reconstructed tongue by repeatedly poking a doppler in his mouth. He was a good sport, and would point which way to go until we heard the pulses. As our residents asked him the same questions day after day, he'd kindly nod and give thumbs up or thumbs down. He'd even wink as I gave him the apologetic look.

Do you have a tongue? Are you able to tell your family that you love them, or share a joke with a friend, or taste your turkey next Thanksgiving? This man, with all that he'd gone through and all that he'd lost, could find a reason to smile each day.

I am certain that we *each* have trials and pet peeves that are unfathomable to other people. But I am equally certain we each have something—at least as much as this man—to be deeply grateful for.

Pediatrics Chose Me

A four-year-old girl, coming out of a visit with me, committed to being a doctor when she grows up.

I had been chatting with her mother about her growth and development, and the little girl was trying to interrupt our discussion. "If you win a game," she said, "you can have *two quarters*!" She held up a stack of pennies. "Are you ready to play the game?"

I told her, "If you hop up on the table, I will play doctor! First I will go wash my hands."

When I came back, she was poised at the edge of the table sitting perfectly still. I handed her a strawberry-flavored tongue blade. She and I took turns looking with the ophthalmoscope and listening with the stethoscope. (However, I did not let her look in my ears for elephants.) Her mother told me it was the first time that she'd ever sat through an entire doctor's visit without screaming.

"You win the game!" I announced. "And you can have a sticker."

"Can we play again? If you win, I will give you *two quarters*!"

I think I did win.

Stickers

A five-year-old boy came in to check on a possible ear infection. He was smiley and very cooperative throughout the exam. He even let me look in his ears twice. I showed him a plastic model of an ear and explained what everything was, and he was fascinated with its parts. He smiled excessively the whole time.

When I was done with the visit, he finally popped the question: "Do you think I can get a sticker today?" Apparently he would agree to any amount of examining as long as he got his sticker.

As we were walking out the door, the doctor glanced over the previous notes in the chart. She paused. "Looks like you guys never came back for your second H1N1 shot?"

The little boy began to cry. He had been told that there would be no shots this visit. Outside, the two nurses quibbled over who would have to deliver the shot.

"I know," I said. "If you will be brave for your shot, we will give you *four* stickers. The *good* kind, out of the special secret drawer. How does that sound?"

The biggest grin spread across his face. He didn't even flinch when he got the needle.

Noah

During a family outing over the holidays, my twelve-year-old brother-in-law, Noah, made a record of sixty-two steps at ice-skating before falling. He has Down's syndrome, and this was the best he could do during his first-ever day on the rink. In the beginning we couldn't peel him away from the walls. When we held his hands, he couldn't even balance well enough to ride along. He was more interested in flopping to the ground and eating the ice. But we told him it was important to get up every time he fell. He was terrified, but we just kept picking him up and setting him on his feet to try again. Within five laps, he went hands-free, showing off with his arms outstretched and shouting "Vector, OH YEAH!" (This is a reference to his favorite movie, *Despicable Me*.)

I started tutoring Noah when he was eight years old, before I applied to medical school. At first I was skeptical whether we would make any progress. He had a limited vocabulary and could not form complete sentences, and I was surprised that he was in a regular classroom where he was learning to read and write along with other kids his age. He was able to write the alphabet though, so I started by giving him all the answers to his homework, letter by letter.

But over time, as I began to understand his slurred speech and became more effective at rephrasing questions, I realized that he actually understood much of what he was being taught. This made working with him more enjoyable, and I became very invested in his success.

I am still constantly surprised by his growth. Now he is thirteen years old and reads at second grade level. He holds long conversations about his favorite movies. He loves to sing and play piano, and his latest trick is writing out pages of music notes as he plays. His most endearing quality, though, is his social awareness. He is jubilant and silly around his siblings, which is delightful to watch. He is also very caring and empathetic. When he sees that I am sad, he gives me a hug and says with a concerned look, "Marie okay? Be happy!"

If a kid with Down's syndrome can do all this, what's to stop *you* from your greatest accomplishment? All people have a great potential to reach for regardless of their limits. I just consider it a great blessing to be able to give people the tools they need to live and function at their best.

My Hunger Diet

My rotations in primary care have driven home one theme: Most things that get you hospitalized and killed could have been prevented with healthy lifestyle changes. And it seems we never hesitate to tell patients what they hate to hear: "Quit smoking. Eat fruits and vegetables. Get off the couch."

Doctors can be truly puzzled by how, even in the face of imminent death, patients act like these changes are dramatic and impossible! Is it really that hard? Why would they rather *die* than walk for five minutes a day?

Well, I was so curious about this rather-die phenomenon, I wanted to try walking those five minutes in the patient's shoes.

So I started what I called the Hunger Diet. It was not scientific in any way, and I don't actually recommend that anyone else try this. I didn't count calories or restrict any food groups or try to lose a lot of weight. I simply ate less than I wanted to at every meal. And I only did it for a limited time so I didn't develop an eating disorder. The only purpose of this exercise was for me to *feel* what my patients felt when I'd tell them they needed to lose weight. You know, because as an Asian who normally eats like it's Thanksgiving at every meal, I fully realize that it's unfair for me to ask other people to deprive themselves when I've never had to.

When I first announced my diet, my mother-in-law shook her head and protested, "But you're not fat at all!" My answer was a cheerful "I agree! But I can't wait until I'm fat. It'll be too late!" She raised a skeptical eyebrow.

I kept it up for about two weeks before switching to a more sustainable diet and exercise program. In the process, I learned some fun things that I'd like to pass on.

1. Hunger *is* a game.

You have to keep playing in order to win. It's a little kid's game, where my opponent's only strategy is to nag persistently. It's a very addicting game: Oh man, it really gets in the way of everything I need to accomplish in life. I kicked my discipline into serious overdrive to ignore the urge to give in. I told myself, "I am going to be hungry at least two hours before the next meal, and that's okay." My body replied, "No, it's *not* okay! Wah!!!"

2. Ignore tantrums.

I saw this as parenting practice. Whenever my hunger would throw a tantrum, I did my best to ignore it. It was easy during the day when I was running around the hospital thinking hard about my patients. It was harder in the evening when I was trying to study before dinner. I ended up doing *more* intense studying, and a few times I even got on the treadmill to pass the time. The idea is to be vigilant and more stubborn than your kid—er, body. When it's hungry, do anything *but* feed it. (Okay, I do not consider that last part to be parenting practice!)

Just remember what they say: Sporadic rewards are the most powerful. If you give in to the tantrum once, you might as well give in every single time.

3. Stock up on negative calories!

I let my guard down a couple times. One day I was woken up from a nap just before dinner. I was so groggy and incoherent, I accidently filled up my plate and ate my usual amount without even thinking. Another day I had a really stressful time at work. I was complaining to my husband throughout dinner, and, again without thinking, I went back for seconds and thirds. Well, it took a while to talk myself out of the guilt that ensued. In the end, it was no big deal—I just got on the treadmill and erased my binges.

This was just a small taste (pun intended,) so why was I sounding so anorexic, schizophrenic, and frankly pathetic? To be honest, it probably would have been easier in many ways if I'd actually calculated calories in and out, because in reality I was probably starving at an unhealthy rate for those couple of weeks. But I did get what I was looking for, which was to tread down this oft-traveled road and gain a sense of what the experience is like *psychologically*.

On the one hand, I can see that a person is not just a box, and losing weight is not a simple matter of inserting less. Every day of a diet is emotional. One's entire self-worth can be tied up in whether or not that great plan was followed correctly. The determination-pride-binge-guilt cycle can be exhausting!

On the other hand, I say no! A person is *nothing but* a box, and losing weight is *quite* a simple matter of inserting less! Why should one make it an emotional mess, when it can just be a plain old chore like paying the phone bill or scrubbing the toilet? What pride? What guilt? Just get down to business!

And on it goes. Bottom line: Staying healthy is both harder and easier than one might imagine. It's a commitment like any other. It's not a cakewalk, but you do have to walk off the cakes you eat!

Death Is Optional! We'll Live Forever! So Far So Good!

Is modern medicine to blame for society feeling this way?

In my twenty-seven years, I've only lost one close friend to cancer. He survived longer than the average person with his disease, but still, I was incredulous when it happened and I couldn't help but feel that the doctors and treatments had failed him. I expected him to live. My grandmother, by the time she was a teenager, had seen nine of her siblings buried.

During my OB rotation, I took part in the deliveries of nineteen babies. Eleven vaginal births and eight C-sections. Nobody died! Everybody went home! Just a hundred years ago, at least two of those babies wouldn't have made it, and chances are I would have watched a mother die in labor too.

Our expectations—and our reality—have come a long way.

I once talked to a professor who volunteered as an ER chaplain. She would help families cope when patients got diagnosed with terminal cancer, or got smashed to pieces, or got their life support pulled. She told me that grieving individuals were prone to asking her, "Is this normal? Am I doing this right?"

No one dies anymore, relatively. Not only that, but on the rare occasion that people do struggle and suffer, they do it quietly, privately. We don't experience it, don't know what death should look like, and certainly don't accept it as a natural part of life—until it happens to someone very close to us, or to ourselves. So the death of a loved one, or even our own, may be the first one we've seen. We haven't been prepared by watching lots of others deal with the same experience, and we frankly don't know how to act.

I hate to report this: Unfortunately, though our road has been paved, lighted, and extended by miles, it still leads to certain death. Many of us, by the time we've reached the end of the scenic route, have forgotten where we were going. Instead of coming gently to a stop, we want to slam the breaks, obstruct oncoming traffic, and flag down highway patrol: "I'm breaking down! SAVE ME!!!"

Is this natural? Is it good? My fear is that, in all this gaining of extra health and life, we may be losing a vital part of our humanity.

A Bill From 3 Months Ago?

As a patient, that is often the extent of my contact with my radiologists. I'm told that no radiologist has ever been recognized at the grocery store by someone shouting, "Hey, that's my doctor!" Some people even think that a radiologist is someone with a two-week certification from the local community college. One might wonder, "Where is the doctorly glory in this desk job?"

And yet, in a little dark cubicle off in the corner of the hospital basement, ALL THE MAGIC OF MEDICINE UNFOLDS!!

Well, at least, that's how the Physics geek in me feels about Radiology. If you are interested in this geekery, read on!

In the earliest stages of medical school, we were taught about clinical problem-solving using simulated patients (i.e., fake patients on the computer.) We would click through the questions we wanted to ask, the physical exam maneuvers, and any tests and imaging we wanted to order. Then we were expected to make the diagnosis and plan the treatment. That was a bit overwhelming at first, and the actual reasoning came slowly, but this exercise taught me one reliable shortcut: The radiologist has all the answers! No matter how confused I felt by the clinical picture, I could usually make the diagnosis by ordering an imaging study and reading the interpretation given by the radiologist.

Of course, good doctors rarely use that shortcut in real life, and the answers are not always readily available to radiologists. The clinical picture is not usually as confusing as it was to me as a first-year medical student, and I can now make many diagnoses based on the patient's story and my exam (shocking!) But a lot of what we know in medicine, we know from imaging. Seeing the pathology is what really confirms what I think I'm dealing with. *Seeing is believing*.

And that's why radiologists are so excited about the advancing technology that has revolutionized medicine again and again. As we build faster computers and higher resolution scanners to give us clearer and clearer images, we are closing the gap of uncertainty. This makes a crucial difference in many cases where the more we know for sure, the better we can tailor the treatment. *Knowledge is power*.

I've always been interested in the nitty-gritty of how the universe works. Perhaps it's not surprising, then, that I found the Radiology textbook to be the best book I've read during medical school. It explained how shadows are translated from densities, and densities from pathology. It explained how to extrapolate the reality of a disease from a two-dimensional image. And the more I read, the more I came to appreciate the order and logic behind what most doctors and medical students dismiss as something for the experts—some even call it "voodoo."

The real magic lies in that order. The shadows are not random; they are purposeful. Within them, the truth is plainly shown to those who understand. I just *love* that!

White Coat Syndrome

At my school, medical students are strictly forbidden from wearing long white coats. This is a big deal, since the coat we wear is supposed to carry a huge and unmistakable distinction. Short coat = medical student (a newbie who doesn't sign orders, doesn't write prescriptions, and is not a legal entity.) Long coat = doctor (the real deal.) We are *never* to mislead our patients by calling ourselves "doctors," acting like we are in charge, or, worst of all, wearing a long white coat.

Oh, but the significance of medical clothing is anything but straightforward. First of all, patients don't always know the long coat/short coat rule. To complicate things, nowadays pharmacists, nurses, dieticians, and other hospital staff often wear white coats of varying lengths (mostly long, probably to spite the medical students.) Then again, many doctors have stopped bothering to wear any coat at all. The net result is that everybody who wears a coat is somewhat important-looking and no one can exactly tell who does what from their clothing, but patients usually assume that all white coats are doctors.

Well, it's not surprising that despite all this fuss over the strict dress code, sometimes I get mistaken for a doctor anyway—and this has really caused *me* some confusion and embarrassment.

Nurses often see me standing behind a counter, and when they address a question to "Doctor," I still find myself turning around, expecting to find a doctor behind me.

Once a resident relayed a compliment to me: "Mr. Jones told me that his 'young doctor' is great!" I just blinked stupidly and asked, "What young doctor?"

Another time, I was assigned to drop off a blood sample at the lab. This being my very first week in the hospital, I stumbled up and down the same hallway several times until someone finally asked if I was lost. I explained that I was looking for the lab but the only entrance I could find was labeled "AUTHORIZED." He gave me this look that conveyed my total idiocy. So then I too looked at myself, and realized that I looked pretty "AUTHORIZED" indeed.

It's gotten better though.

Towards the end of my third year, someone I met in the ER introduced me to all the doctors that walked by, telling them I was with Family Medicine. I thought he was just being friendly. He was floored to find out I was a medical student, and immediately stopped making further introductions. I pointed out the obvious short coat, and he said, "Oh, of course! But you seemed so confident, I didn't even look at that!"

Eventually I took the coat so much for granted that sometimes I would forget to leave it in the car as I trudged into ordinary civilian places, like the bank or the grocery store. I suppose I must have looked like a real presumptuous jerk. Who knows, maybe I even got featured in The People of Walmart?

I won't lie; it's been a pretty big transformation. Slowly but steadily my classmates and I have been growing into the short white coats. I can't tell you how terrifying it is that we'll be growing out of them so inevitably soon!

From Speed Dating to Wedding Day

From September to March of fourth year, I was a contestant in The Match—the process by which residency programs and applicants find each other. The name aptly recalls the feel of a dating game show.

I started by filling out my profile at the match website, taking care to highlight all of my strengths and downplay any weaknesses. Then I browsed all the profiles of programs and coughed up a hefty fee to contact the ones I found attractive. Meanwhile, the programs were receiving hundreds of solicitations from others all over the world.

In the next round, I waited by the phone. Every time the mail icon popped up with "Invitation to Interview," I would drop everything and find a quiet place to pull out my map and calendar. To make this much more scandalous than it would have otherwise been, I was doing a visiting internship in a specialty other than the one I was courting, and I didn't dare let anyone there know about my two-timing (more on that later.)

My date book was getting pretty full and new invitations kept coming every week. Meanwhile, I enjoyed getting ready for my first interview trip, especially the part where I got to upgrade my wardrobe.

Then came three exciting months of back-to-back visits to hospitals all over the country. From October to January, I averaged one flight leg per weekday, zigzagging from New York to California to Vermont to Texas. (Despite my best efforts to piggyback the east coast interviews, I visited New England five separate times.) At each institution, I had just a few hours to both gain and make an impression. Most of these days consisted of a series of fifteen-minute interviews with several different faculty members—hence, "speed dating."

Some principles of dating apply to these interviews. For example, one shouldn't ask a girl her bra size during the first date. Likewise, it would be foolish for an applicant to ask the faculty directly about the salary and benefits package. Other principles do not apply. For example, one shouldn't let on that one knows too much about one's date, lest one appear stalkerish. On the contrary, having done thorough research shows off an applicant's sincere interest in a program, and vice versa. Well, some interviewers tried to make it a "blind date" by conducting the interview without bothering to look at my application, but that didn't go over well. Just as program directors don't appreciate reciting their website, I don't appreciate reciting my personal statement.

I was extremely giddy hopping off the last plane in mid-January: In just another couple months, I would be "married" (matched!) Of course, I wouldn't know which candidate I'd get until the "wedding day" (match day.) I just hoped it would be an arrangement that my husband could also be happy with.

My final task was the Rank Order List, which boiled down to crunching a lot of numbers and thinking deeply about pros and cons. We made a huge spreadsheet to rank the programs based on quality of education, location, and lifestyle factors such as availability of sword practice groups and proximity of Asian groceries. Surprisingly, this part was straightforward and non-controversial for us. I was blessed with so many great options, I really would have been happy anywhere.

Ultimately, my fate was handed over to a computer in Washington, D.C. This part diverges from the traditional job hunt story: Every year, each residency program and each applicant compiles a list of potential matches in order of preference, the computer makes The Match, and the end result is that each applicant gets accepted to exactly one or zero residencies.

The match algorithm, though supposedly error-proof, is a secret. This naturally keeps everyone on their superstitious toes. Last-minute calls and emails were exchanged between programs and applicants, saying, "You're my number one!" Attention from your program of choice is very nice, while the same from a less-desirable place comes off as desperate. In the end, I don't think any of these exchanges affected anyone's ranking one whit. But it sure is flattering to receive some compliments anyway.

There was a gap of about a month between the time we submitted the final rank list and the time our matches were unveiled. In this period, I second-guessed my ability to match every single day. Even though the magic number was about ten interviews to guarantee a match, it became my husband's full-time job to reassure me that I was not the one-in-a-thousand loser who couldn't appeal to even one of seventeen programs. Theoretically, that could have happened if I'd systematically offended all hundred or so people that I'd interviewed with. But okay, it was just a tad dramatic.

March 15th was Match Day. I called it the Ides of Match. I came to the celebration in my wedding shoes. Our families were gathered for the occasion. Speeches were given by important people. Breakfast was served. I was shaking from head to toe and staring at my watch. My brother-in-law asked if I had any feeling about where I would go, and all I could say was, "I am confident in how I made my rank list. Whatever I get will be the best that I could have done." For all I knew, that could have been number seventeen, or even number eighteen (in the wrong specialty.)

At 9:00 sharp, I struggled to get through the throng of classmates to find the envelope with my name on it. I brought it back to where my family was gathered. For a moment I couldn't decipher any of the words dancing off the page. And then it caught me: "Dartmouth... DARTMOUTH!!!!" I was surrounded by a frenzy of hugs and laughs and tears.

Six months of hopes, doubts, and gallons of adrenaline! Dartmouth was my very favorite program. Who knew that this madness we jokingly call a dating service would actually land me exactly where I am supposed to be?

A Honeymoon

For reasons now elusive to me, I thought it would be a good idea to get married *two days* before the start of medical school. I also micromanaged the whole production, from Photoshopping invitations to drawing the cake design to making frosting flowers to scanning albums for the slideshow to frying crêpes. In the day between the wedding and the first day of school, my husband and I hosted an extended family gathering at our new house. I remember thinking, "If I can pull off this wedding, I can totally handle medical school!"

The ensuing four months of brutal book beating cast some doubt on my invincibility. That first semester, when people asked how I was holding up, I would say, "Well, med school isn't exactly a honeymoon."

During the school year, I spent most of my waking hours locked in a study room on campus with a dedicated group of classmates. I had to compromise many of the things that normal people would take for granted. My husband did all of the cooking because menu-planning was too stressful for me. The only chores I could take on were things that I could afford to neglect. I considered a "date" to be the half-hour I allocated to eating dinner every night. Saying no to extended family functions became a reflex. I learned to laugh rather than take offense when people suggested that I try to achieve some sort of "work-life balance" by doing more of whatever they wanted me to do—they simply didn't understand that I needed less work and not more life.

How was this situation ever made possible? What kind of man would marry into this situation, taking a medical student for a bride and medical school for a honeymoon? Someone who is very supportive and patient and adaptable to change. Someone slightly crazy. And, yeah, perhaps someone you should feel a little sorry for.

It wasn't a conventional newlywed life. Instead of easing into a charming little game of house, we were confronted right away with all the realities of adulthood. Medical school created its own marital problems: A medical student is always on the verge of a crisis, at least once a week according to the exam schedule, and the looming crisis usually demands some earth-shattering sacrifice on the part of the spouse (which is perhaps why so many couples end up divorced during these years.) But it was a valuable team-building experience, one that strengthened our relationship much more than a relaxing two-week cruise would have. We gained big skills. We even found a silver lining to our initial difficulties.

An important one is time management. I'm convinced now that time management is all there is to life. The reason this skill is such a big perk in a spouse is that it essentially magnifies how much spouse you have. With proper management, "time off" can seem everlasting. During the summer between first and second year, it felt like I got to do everything I'd ever wanted to in life, including working full-time and lounging around as a housewife on the side. I cleaned house every day, I made lots of crafts, I baked, I canned, I scrapbooked endlessly. I even carried on these activities into the next school year.

And I don't mean to make it sound like we never had *any* honeymoon. In the last three years, we've made good use of our vacations and trotted all over the globe. We've visited China, the Dominican Republic, Singapore, Italy, France, England, Jersey, Scotland, and Puerto Rico. We've moved for short periods to Las Vegas, Sacramento, and San Francisco. We've enjoyed weekend trips to Houston, New Orleans, Chicago, and New England.

There is no reason that having a career should hinder having a life, and no reason it should require someone else to drop everything. All these experiences have united us in the effort to rise above adversity. That's what made these four years a great honeymoon.

Zigzagging

Interview season was probably my favorite rotation in medical school. Every day I found myself in a new city with a new opportunity. Previous students had warned me that the novelty would wear off, and that I would get fed up enough to cancel a bunch of interviews. Fortunately, I actually couldn't get enough! I looked at it this way: If I could be happy every single day in Surgery, notwithstanding getting up at 4 AM and holding retractors for hours at a time, what's not to love about fancy dinners in black suits and high heels?

Except for a few jetlagged early morning rounds, I really wouldn't have traded this experience for the world—for the simple reason that our country is so quirky! Look at how my horizons have expanded in three short months!

Worcester, Massachusetts:
They call it "Woostah." Man, I thought people had problems pronouncing "Nevada" correctly.

Galveston, Texas:
I was told that overachievers wouldn't fit in too well with the extremely laid-back "islander" culture. Never mind that this is still Texas and the island is connected to the mainland by several highway bridges.

Providence, Rhode Island:

When asking for directions, expect references to landmarks and structures that *used to be there*. Just take a left at the old interstate and keep going until you see that empty lot where Dunkin' Donuts used to be. In other words, next time just bring your GPS!

Danville, Pennsylvania:

A rich widow decided to blow her husband's life savings on building a huge, high-quality academic hospital in the middle of a 5,000 population town—just imagine Mayo Clinic doing its thing in Duckwater, Nevada. More than one patient has arrived at the hospital in a horse and buggy.

New Orleans:

If someone asks you what you did this weekend, the answer is "I ate at ___ Restaurant, and I ordered ___." If you say something like, "I saw the president at ___ Restaurant," the follow-up question is still going to be, "So what'd you order?"

San Francisco:

If you don't turn your wheels enough while parked, you will get a ticket. If you don't give up your seat for an old person on the bus, you will get a ticket. If you don't bring your own grocery bags, you will be charged ten cents a bag. But you can be nude in public, as long as you bring something to sit on.

El Paso, Texas:

The annual snowstorm occurred the day before my interview. Flights were cancelled. Taxis were scarce. Businesses were closed. Nobody was expected to make it to work. I bought a last-minute ticket on the only flight daring enough to land, and was greeted by a treacherous half inch of snow.

Burlington, Vermont:

Ben & Jerry's ice cream was founded here. Or maybe it was actually *found* here, occurring naturally during the -30 degree winter. Also, Canadian flags are flown alongside American flags.

Medical School Is Not a Hobby

I am graduating with some fantastic doctors. I've worked closely with many of my classmates over the years, and I've seen them in some shining moments. I'm ever impressed when attendings grill them with difficult questions and they get the right answers without batting an eye. I'm proud of how diligently they take care of patients, listening at length to get all the details of the story, pouring over medical records and evidence-based articles to tailor the best treatment plan. In six years, if I am back in Reno after completing residency, I hope to see many of them practicing in the community.

I've also had the privilege this year of teaching a group of second-year medical students in a "doctoring skills" class. These kids are just about to embark on their clinical years, the adventure that my class has just completed. They are motivated and brilliant! When I first met them, they hadn't been taught many of the mechanical aspects of practicing medicine, like how to properly document a patient visit. Over the course of the semester, they improved by leaps and bounds. When I read their final reports at the end of the semester, they blew me away with their attention to detail and understanding of the big picture. Wow.

I call my second-year students "kids" because I feel like a grandmother to them; because the weeks have felt like years, I look back on their time through "aged" eyes. But teaching them has also kept me young! It's refreshing to share in their excitement about the future, and to remember how far we have come.

Four years ago, my class hadn't taken up medicine yet. Many of us were just wrapping up our undergraduate work or leaving other careers. Though we all had a science background, I personally hadn't taken any Anatomy classes; I knew there were arms and legs and torsos, I didn't know the spleen was a real organ.

What were you doing four years ago? Say for a minute that you took up a new hobby, like figure-skating. How would that sport be coming along, four years later? Since you're here and reading this, I think we can assume you haven't skated into and been crushed under a Zamboni. That's lucky. Imagine that time when you were practicing outdoors, and the ice crumbled beneath your skates, and you fell headfirst into a lake. Did that hypothetical experience teach you not to skate on frozen lakes? Ah, then you are theoretical proof that immersion is an effective way to learn. Or would that be osmosis?

Just like that, four years gone by so fast! What does figure-skating have to do with medical school? Both can hurt your brains. In figure-skating, keeping your brains intact *depends on* your competence. In medical school, keeping your brains intact *determines* your competence.

Finally, a few facts* and statistics to debunk the misinformation you've been given by the media about the medical profession. Don't be intimidated by the brandishing of knives and needles. Deep down inside, doctors are really just a bunch of sissies who like to play House. Take a moment to reflect on this before reading on.

Fact: By the end of medical education, the average graduate has memorized 14,853 pages of textbook information, and forgotten the equivalent of 35,688 pages. (How is this possible? Well, for every Histology slide we memorize, we forget several childhood memories.)

Fact: During one semester of Pathology class, the studious medical student contracts no less than fifteen incurable diseases. The proper medical term for this is "hypochondriasis," but some consider being a hypochondriac to be a good survival strategy. That's why we must be ever vigilant in our own medical care. You never know when you'll get diagnosed with a brain tumor—after you insist on getting your blood sugars and cholesterol checked—for the third time this month.

Fact: Despite being in 19th grade, medical students still get treated like kindergarteners. Consider, for example, the exam conditions. Exam-taking requires juice boxes in the form of 5-hour energy drinks every hour, and snack time. Absolutely no bathroom breaks are allowed without a chaperone.

Colleagues of the Class of 2013: Congrats! Future patients of the Class of 2013: Try not to get sick on July 1st.

*Not actual facts.

3

DOCTORS vs. PATIENTS

TV once made me believe that doctors and patients had a hero-damsel relationship. Social media now tells me that doctors are a last resort. To be truthful, this is a difficult topic for me to write about, but one that I can't avoid bringing up. In order for us to be on the same team—and health is really a team effort—we need to try on each other's shoes. In the first half of this section, I lay out my shoes for you. In the second half, I try on yours.

People Need Oil Changes Too

While juggling a dozen medications for a patient with diabetes, high blood pressure, and high cholesterol, the doctor suggested, "I'd like to draw a few labs to monitor the effects of your medications. It's been over a year, and I can't keep giving you these drugs without knowing if they're working."

"I can't, doctor," replied the patient. "I lost my insurance. Whatever the cost is of these labs, I don't have that money." His wife bit her lip.

The doctor and patient exchanged a few rounds of explanations. I thought, *He will never convince this guy to pay for the labs.*

The doctor abruptly changed the subject: "Do you have a car?"

The patient was taken aback. "Yeah, I drive a truck."

"Do you get the oil changed?"

"Yes, every time."

"Do you wait until the car breaks down before you get an oil change?"

"No."

The doctor turned to me as he heard me chuckle. "Where am I going with this, Marie?"

With a grin, I asked, "Would you like to have a heart attack, or would you like to prevent it?"

The patient and his wife exchanged looks of alarm. "Prevent it!"

The doctor nodded. "Then I'm telling you, you need these labs."

I know from too many personal experiences that health care can be expensive. So can housing, food, gas, vacationing, and having an iPhone. We all choose our own priorities, of course, but you can't do any of the other things if you're not alive.

Life and Death

A two-week-old infant was brought to the Pediatrician's office for the first time. The new parents were tired, but ambitious to get it right. Dr. X examined the baby and happily reported that he was healthy and thriving. She went on to chat with the parents about how they were adjusting, what to expect, what precautions to take. The parents were eagerly jotting down notes.

A seven-year-old was next on the schedule. Dr. X hadn't seen this kid since he had laryngitis two years ago, and probably wouldn't see him again until the next time he was sick (at a certain point, children start skipping their well visits.) Today he was sent from school because he had pink eye, and the school would not let him return unless he had antibiotics. Our exam suggested he had viral conjunctivitis, but, for the sake of his continued education, Dr. X wrote for the antibiotics.

At thirteen, the next patient was steadily climbing off the growth chart. A long discussion was had about the need to exercise daily, cut down on sugary beverages, and eat vegetables instead of fast food. The family expressed no intention to follow any of this counsel unless it would be convenient.

Pediatricians spend entire visits discussing vaccinations and antibiotics, obesity and anorexia, medications and asymptomatic life-threatening conditions. Eventually they pass the baton to their Adult colleagues.

A thirty-five-year-old man came to the Family Medicine clinic for a checkup required by his new employer. This was his first doctor's visit since he was a kid on his parents' health insurance plan. He was proud to say he'd always been healthy. He had never been told he had dangerously high blood pressures.

A sixty-four-year-old woman with lung cancer called 911 when she felt suddenly short of breath. When the paramedics arrived, she insisted on finishing her cigarette before entering the ambulance.

One of the most rewarding aspects of working with children is having the ability to guide young patients in making healthy lifelong choices and habits. One of the most frustrating aspects of working with adults is being held suddenly responsible for the aftermath of a lifetime of poor lifestyle choices. It seems like people travel down a slippery slope between being born to super-parents to ultimately not caring whether they live or die.

How to Win Friends and Influence Doctors

There was a patient who made a huge impression on me the first day that we met. He was a diabetic who'd let himself go, had multiple amputations, and was now undergoing a long course of treatment for widespread infections. He knew he wouldn't live much longer when our team visited him.

We were led by a well-respected physician, one that I'd known throughout my training as exemplifying competence and bedside etiquette. When this doctor started to explain the plan, the patient became hostile, hurling insults and profanities. "My surgeon told me the opposite! What you say doesn't count. You're just the University doctor."

The doctor nodded quietly and continued to listen as the patient ranted about the surgeon, the infectious disease specialist, the nurses, the lack of communication, and other problems of the American health care system. Finally, he deescalated to asking how long our doctor had been living in Reno. "You see! I knew you weren't from here! I've lived here for fifty-five years, and you and I both know that what they're doing ain't right!"

Within days, he became like a vegetable. But until then, every day of his remaining life, this man made a dogged effort to burn all his bridges with the medical staff.

This is the part where I would like to say that his demeaning attitude did not affect the quality of his medical care, that we were just as concerned about him as we would have been about a sweet old lady who brought us cookies. But that would be a blatant lie. And this is hard for me to accept, at this stage of my training. I *want* us to be impartial. I *want* us to uphold the exact same standard for everyone.

But we are human, after all. And the doctor-patient relationship is a *relationship.* Don't get me wrong, this guy had his meals brought, blood pressures checked, labs drawn, wound dressings changed. Actually, a great many extra hours were spent trying to figure out how to deal with him. It just could have been a better experience for everyone involved.

Being human, we can also be influenced to provide better care. That's why most of the time, we are *encouraged* to practice medicine with "humanity." Caring about our patients motivates us to go that extra mile.

From my observations, the best patients seem to know exactly how to maximize their benefit from our humanity.

For one, good patients recognize that we are human beings, and treat us as such. I guess it can be hard for people to see their doctors as more than white coats, just as it can be hard for us to see our patients as more than diagnoses. We do presume that our patients are people outside of medicine, and we are too! We like jokes and insights. We like to hear about hobbies or major life events. But those who act like a doctor is "just the check-up person" (as one girl put it,) probably don't get much other than annual prescriptions. Looking back on my own writing, the patients who really stood out have had a sense of humor and a positive outlook. They were able to teach me about overcoming adversity.

Good patients also treat us like their allies. And rightly so, because I sure came to medical school with the intention of helping people! Bad outcomes do happen, but believe it or not, it's not because the doctors are trying to kill people. Demonizing and alienating us usually will not make us sympathize. In fact, when new patients come ranting about the list of doctors they're in the process of suing, I think doctors are more likely to distance themselves. Like everyone else, doctors are more willing to keep trying when our best efforts are acknowledged and appreciated. That is not to say that patients should never complain, but that they should try to make it constructive.

Perhaps most importantly, good patients pull their own weight. There's a reason we all *love* patients who exercise, eat healthy, stay on top of their meds, and generally heed our advice. It's because, as surprising as it may sound, doctors are not "health care." Patients are. It is each individual's job to maintain their own health, to do the right things from day to day. Doctors only help to bridge the gap when something falls apart—I call this "sick care." So it's great when patients ask questions, study it out and make conscientious decisions, and commit to healthy lifestyles. (It's even okay for patients to tell us about the "alternative medicine" they're using, so long as they spare us the lecture about how marijuana and essential oils are superior to modern medicine.) It is validating and reassuring when patients try to show us that they care about their health—because if they don't care, why should we?

Delirium at 83

Hospital care seen through the eyes of a delirious patient.

My bottle of pills was taken away from me. The nurse came and yanked them right out from underneath me, with that awful smile and falsely reassuring me, "You won't be needing these anymore, Haley."

I was devastated. "You can't do this to me," I protested, "You don't know what it's like!"

My small daughter, Shannon, looked up from beside the bed. "What's wrong, Mommy?"

I'd forgotten that she was standing right there. "Oh, nothing, Honey. Don't worry about it." I put my arm around her protectively.

In the distance, I heard someone say, "Grandma, you're talking to Shannon again; she's dead. Those pills were making you crazy." I searched into the dark room for this new voice, and my eyes settled on someone I'd never seen before.

"Who are you?" I asked suspiciously.

The stranger winced. "I'm Sarah, your granddaughter. You don't remember me?" She stepped closer and put a hand on my shoulder.

I looked from this person to the anxious little girl beside my bed, my three-year-old daughter. *I don't have a granddaughter, I'm twenty-eight! What kind of sick game is this?* I panicked. "Nurse? NURSE!!" I shrieked.

The nurse came running frantically back, but ignoring me, she turned directly to the stranger. "Is she getting agitated again?" The stranger, "Sarah," nodded.

"*Me,* agitated?!" I cried. I was becoming furious with this whole ridiculous situation. "First you take away my pain medication without my consent, and not a minute later you've let this bum teenager wander into my room! Aren't you supposed to take care of me? You people are incompetent! You all deserve to be fired!"

The nurse had gone into the hall. I could hear her voice mumbling. "Patient in 516... agitated. She's been... now hallucinating and talking to dead relatives. Should I give her...? Okay. Thank you, Doctor."

The stranger continued to stand in the corner, looking terrified. "Grandma, please stop this," she begged.

I was so fed up. And so helpless. "I don't know who you are! Get out of my room!" She didn't move. I threw my milk carton in her direction. She took a step back, but didn't leave. "GET OUT!!!!" I threw my fork, my pudding, and the rest of the trash off my dinner tray. Then I threw the tray. She finally backed out.

Several uniformed men burst in. The harsh lights flashed on. One of them grabbed my arm. I thrashed wildly about and yelled "NO! STOP! LET ME GO!!" I could feel my throat burning. The others took hold of my legs and together they tied all of my limbs to the bed. I continued to thrash, shaking my IV pole. But it was no use. I broke down sobbing.

The nurse marched in triumphantly. Before I realized to resist, she attached a syringe to my IV line and pushed the injection.

Slowly, slowly, the room turned dark.

Holiday ER Stunt

As a fascinating holiday stunt, I spent Christmas Eve in the ER—as a patient.

After signing all the paperwork and explaining my situation, my husband and I were asked to find a seat and wait for my name to be called. The waiting room was pretty empty. Before we'd even agreed on where to sit, my name was called.

Someone took my vitals, and saw that I was not going to die. When asked again, I stuck to my story.

"Fast service!" My husband commented.

"That was just triage," I told him. "The real waiting begins now."

"But at least they got you through triage fast!"

"Umm, I've already triaged myself. That's why I'm here in the first place."

A lady was sobbing loudly. A man was pacing frantically and occasionally moaning in agony. A volunteer was apologetically offering blankets. I opened a textbook and got to work.

Two hours later, I'd reviewed the textbook chapters pertaining to my condition, decided on the course of action I would take as the ER physician, and also made several attempts to set a new record for Fruit Ninja. About a dozen other people had since arrived and been called in. I went up to the triage desk again.

A couple was yelling at the triage nurse and threatening never to come back again. When the nurse finished dealing with them, she turned to me with a very exasperated look and asked, "Can I help you?"

I tried a different approach. With a smile and a casual tone, I said, "I just wanted to get a rough idea of where I am on the list."

She scanned for my name. "You are at the top! I have you on the fast track, but there aren't very many beds turning around."

"Wow, really? I've been here for two hours."

"You will probably be the next person called. But we also get heart attacks and strokes," she explained. Of course, I knew all too well.

Another hour later, after several more people fast-tracked past me, I was brought into a room in the pediatrics ER, which I knew served as overflow for when the main ER was full. It was freezing, and I had to change from my winter clothes into a thin gown. I was given one small warmed blanket, which quickly lost its heat. I huddled into the blanket and asked my husband to pile on several extra sheets from the cabinet. After pressing all the levers, I gave up trying to raise the back of the bed, so I stayed lying flat, bundled, craning my neck to watch the TV in the corner of the room.

In another hour, the doctor came in to make his initial evaluation. He laughed when he saw me, but was kind enough to bring several more hot blankets. He asked me again what happened. As a courtesy, he listened to my heart and lungs. He told me the list of tests he wanted to run, instructed me not to eat or drink anything in case I had to go for surgery, and then disappeared for another hour.

The nurse finally came back to put in an IV and draw my blood. A really sick baby had arrived just after me, and the doctor had been too busy to write orders for any of my tests.

My husband wondered out loud how much longer we might be there. It had been five hours, and we were just gathering the first, most basic of the studies. The nurse said, best-case scenario, another three hours. I knew that I wouldn't be staying overnight or going for surgery, but that it would be late evening before all the tests were collected. I asked him to call home and tell the family not to wait on us for Christmas Eve dinner.

So this is probably a typical ER day for any given patient: boring, exhausting, uncomfortable, and inefficient. And I might add that those IVs are ridiculously itchy! I can only imagine that patients *without* medical degrees must find it excruciatingly frustrating to wait and suffer. Most of the patients probably don't know what's going on, what's being suspected or tested for, how serious it is, or even whether or not they are going to die.

I've worked these shifts, and I've treated patients like me. It's *not* inefficient from the other side of the door. I know those ER docs are running around frantically on a day like this, constantly seeing new patients, doing procedures, running codes, writing notes and entering orders, calling consultants, following up on results, reassessing, reassuring. In fact, I have never seen an ER doc take a lunch or dinner break no matter which shift they were working.

There is such a difference between what the patient experiences and what the doctor experiences! I feel slightly embarrassed by it, almost like I need to apologize. I'm sure it's hard to take your doctors seriously when they're running in and out and making you wait for hours in between. It's really hard to convey just how much work there is to be done, how much there is to think of, between those hectic runs into the patient room. I don't know how we can close this gap. But at the very least, I want to say this, in case no one else ever does: Your doctors care a lot about your well-being and work really hard for you, even when it doesn't seem like it.

4

ORIGINS AND DESTINATIONS

This is where I finally explain where I came from, why I chose medicine, and how I became the happiest person I know.

A Tiger's Parents

I was born in 1986, the year of the Tiger, to two young doctors in China. My background story would be incomplete without a discussion of my parents and their legacy of excellence in medicine.

My mom graduated from Xiangya Medical School in 1982, as part of the first class of students allowed back to higher education after the Cultural Revolution in China. As an OB for thirteen years, she delivered thousands of babies—dozens daily at about forty cents apiece. In 1990, when I was four, she won the Hunan Province "Housewife of the Decade" competition for her cooking, sewing, crafting, and home decorating.

When she came home from work, after being on call overnight, she would spend her midday nap time reading me stories. When my Yamaha keyboard broke down (repeatedly,) she would bike to the repair shop carrying the keyboard on her back, and then carry the bike up six flights of stairs to our apartment. When I brought home my English homework, which neither of us understood, she would sit with me and look up every single word in the dictionary.

To this day, she cooks, cleans, and drives my sisters all over town to golf practices and music rehearsals, in addition to supporting my dad in his career and working a full-time job herself. And she also comes running to kill off the spiders when my sisters scream for help.

My dad is the man my mom met and fell in love with in medical school over thirty years ago, when they were both in their late teens.

He is the man who sacrificed a color TV to buy me a keyboard when I wanted music lessons, and, when his work shoes were worn through, held off on buying a new pair so I could have my first pair of ice skates. I didn't know it at the time, but he also racked up $1000 in international long-distance phone bills monthly so I could sing him the songs I learned in preschool.

He is the man who, when I just started learning English, would spend hours translating Dr. Seuss books and teaching me the difference between "to," "too," and "two." He also was the first to teach me about physics when I was little, which has turned out to be one of the greatest fascinations of my life.

He is the man who has shown incredible love and patience even when I didn't always believe his life lessons, and continued support even when I chose to make my own paths. This was the greatest gift he ever gave me (besides maybe the brains *and* killer looks,) and one I'll be sure to pass on to my own kids.

And of course, this man would not be who he is, if he were not constantly telling terrible Dad jokes, especially while giving Pharmacology lectures at my medical school. I thanked him later when his mnemonics earned me no less than 4 questions on my USMLE Step 1 exam.

It was for me that these two left their careers in China to pursue a better life in North America. It was also for me, the lonely child that I was at the time, that they produced my two baby sisters whom I love so much—so it can be said that it was for me that they are now faced with the daunting task of parenting teenage daughters all over again.

My parents have always been overly considerate in their efforts to provide for me. My words are inadequate to express my appreciation, to my mom for showing me how womanhood is done, and to my dad for all that he's sacrificed and all that he is. I am so proud to be their daughter.

Roadmaps

I should tell you what attracted me to medicine. Most immediately, it was my violin teacher. No, he isn't in the business of churning out doctors. He just did a really good job teaching me to play violin.

Growing up as the only child (for ten years) of two doctors, people would ask me if I wanted to be a doctor, and I would say, "Umm, NO!" I rather wanted to rebel from this "destiny" of mine. Actually, I always thought I could make it as a musician. My parents started me on piano when I was tiny. Later I took violin and voice lessons, and was heavily involved in orchestras and choirs throughout high school and college. I was encouraged by the strides I made and the feedback I got. On tough days, this is something I still wonder about. Of course, I now recognize that being a professional musician would be a long shot. But, ironically, it was just what I needed to set me in the right trajectory.

My violin teacher was the one who pointed out how my passion for music translates into an aptitude for medicine. He loved to tell me, "If you were a brain surgeon and you missed by *that* much, you would have just killed your patient!" He would then pick up my finger and replace it in the correct place, only a millimeter from where it was before. At the time I couldn't believe there existed perceptible differences that small. But he said many times, "You will be that nit-picky. You will practice the same stupid scale a thousand times until every note is perfect every time. It's not just violin, it's a whole *mentality*. And it will translate into everything you do. You will be the only one on your tennis team who hits against the wall with the same stroke for hours day after day. You will be the brain surgeon I can trust with my life." Sure enough, after years of practicing with that perfectionist mentality, I too became bothered by differences of just millimeters. Eventually he deemed me "suitable for brain surgery," and from then on, that was all I wanted to do.

I think a lot about how lives are changed, and about the people who are in a position to change them. It may not have been what he intended, but I can attribute a great portion of my future life-saving capacity to my violin teacher.

My story is full of these little moments, where someone, at the right time, said something that tweaked the direction I was headed. Most of us take a meandering path, after all.

It's scary, in a way: You or I could, inadvertently, unknowingly, give someone the push they need in the direction of "the rest of their lives." It doesn't matter who you are. It often doesn't even matter your relation to that person. What matters is what they need to hear. You can't plan it. You may not ever know it. But maybe you already did it today. **Never underestimate *your* power to change someone's life.**

Carpe Every Single Diem!

I take a *very* go-getter approach to personal happiness. Granted, my life is great. (It especially seems so if you mostly know me through my writing.) But just like everyone else, I definitely have "those" moments, days, and even weeks. In fact, if you ask a random graduating medical student, they may tell you it's been "one of those" past four years.

"Those" moments don't tend to make good essays to inspire the world. But trust me, I *haven't* edited them out of my life story. You want proof? Here are a few additional snapshots from my first six clinical months:

...It is 3 PM on a Saturday. It is my 33rd hour at the hospital, and my 7th hour standing in the OR holding a pair of retractors. "I know you are post-call," the chief resident had said, "but if you stay for this, it will be the coolest surgery you have ever seen." So far, all I can see is the surgeon poking instruments down a deep, dark hole in the patient. He points and mumbles about structures, but I can't see any of them. I did study up on my anatomy in case he's in the mood for quizzing, but he's not. I shift my weight constantly as my knees are killing me. I watch the clock for a while. I nod off and close my eyes. And all the while, I'm still holding the retractors perfectly still. But what I take away is this: "Life After Getting Your Face Chopped Off" (p.42)

...Halloween at the Trauma Bay. One patient shot himself in the head, another in the chest. A week ago, I had never seen anybody die. Now, I've lost count of how many deaths I've seen. One of the suicidal patients, upon being resuscitated, immediately begins shouting profanities at the medical staff for extending his misery. I begin to question what a doctor is supposed to contribute to a patient's life: "Trauma, Death, and the Big Picture" (p.9)

...I've been working two whole minutes, and the patient I've been assigned has already accused me of trying to poison her, made racist comments to me, and tried to inflict physical injury on me from across the room. "It's not me," I tell myself, "she's schizophrenic." I've made it over two years without struggling to establish rapport with a single patient, and my perfect record ends with this: "How to Say Hello to a Crazy Person" (p.33)

I can see how in the midst of every single stupid day, we may not enjoy being told to "enjoy every moment." And I've also had times when I've been absolutely miserable with everything I've ever dreamed of—things like a big house, an amazing husband, and a prestigious career. Trust me, there is nothing about having everything we want that *makes* us happy. Happiness is not about the situation that surrounds us, but rather the lens through which we choose to see it.

Every day when I wake up, I tell myself, "You will love today. You *will* love today." This may or may not be preceded by me flinging my alarm clock across the room.

A Season For All Things

I have always told people that I know the secret to happiness: *Don't view anything as a means to an end*. You have to see the value of everything you do and endorse every step of it. You have to live in the moment.

I still said this the day I shipped my husband off to Scotland to get his master's degree. It was Labor Day weekend, and I wouldn't see him again until Christmas.

We knew this day would come. We looked forward to it with excitement and dread. He first brought up the idea before we were married, before I was in medical school. I was immediately on board. We both wanted advanced degrees, and I knew that four years was an awful long time for him to wait around for me. We are no strangers to distance. For the first three years of our courtship, we attended universities on opposite ends of the continent. We knew this would be hard, but we knew that we of all people could make it work.

Let's be honest. Long-distance relationships suck, especially in the very beginning. I missed snuggling. I hadn't had to cook or shop for groceries in over two years, and I didn't think I knew how anymore. I was used to having a constant dialogue about our experiences and thoughts—it's my favorite way to bond. But we were on an eight-hour time difference with less than an hour of overlapping free time each day.

Looking back, I truly have to say, I have never regretted this decision. We chose this together when we were both rational and future-oriented. I am so proud of my husband for making this great sacrifice and for doing something good with his life instead of idling away while waiting for me to complete my education. This was the opportunity of a lifetime. I knew he would have wonderful experiences that would strengthen him and our family. He learned to be more disciplined and I learned to be more patient—both will help us to be better prepared for life and parenting.

Over the preceding seven years, we had endured countless trials together and had built a very strong relationship. We knew we were better prepared for this now than we ever were before, and probably more than we ever would be again (since we don't have children right now.)

And with that knowledge, I could be happy. Not only with this process as a means to an end. Not only when I would think of Christmas or next September. I was happy *in the moment* because we were doing our part to move forward with the plan. I was glad that we would be together again, but I couldn't afford to make myself miserable by focusing on his absence. So I continued my third-year medical student life, keeping myself busy by helping other people, engaging in my duties, and learning all that I could. I was actually kind of grateful for all the extra time I had to study without feeling guilty. I also was able to keep our room totally clean and organized every single day.

And guess what? A year later, he came back, dissertation completed and degree in hand—he'd graduated with distinction! And he wasted no time in unpacking his suitcases and spreading his stuff out all over the floor—a happy sight and a very worthwhile compromise for having a husband.

We never know what life will bring us each day. All we can guarantee is that we will do our best to make it count.

5

THE PROTAGONIST IS A RADIOLOGIST?!

Choosing a specialty is the question of a lifetime for medical students. It pretty much drove me crazy. And maybe when you learn that I chose Radiology, you will assume that I have gone crazy. Please read on: I promise it all makes sense.

An Explanation

One night, months or years ago, my husband looked up from a collection of short stories he was reading, and said, "This one is interesting. The protagonist is a radiologist."

To this, I laughed out loud. "Why would the protagonist be a radiologist?"

Judging by the lukewarm reactions I've received this year when I've told people that I was going into Radiology, I suppose most people feel the same way I did: that there is nothing interesting about a radiologist.

Don't get me wrong, I absolutely adore Radiology and honestly feel that I've made the best possible career choice. But, given that my interest in Radiology did sneak up on me at the last minute after I'd already changed my mind half a dozen times between other specialties, perhaps I owe everyone an explanation.

In the beginning, as I've mentioned, my intention was to be a neurosurgeon. I never felt like it would give me the life I envisioned, but the work sounded challenging and heroic, and that was what brought me to medical school. I quickly realized that being away from my family for 120 hours a week was even less tolerable than I imagined. The neurosurgeons I met on my Surgery rotation, though very nice, made it clear to me that working one-third time (a normal 40-hour workweek) was not acceptable, even for a woman. In fact, I got the impression that having ovaries was entirely incongruent with Neurosurgery—people simply didn't make time for babies and lives in that field. A Surgery resident gave me this valuable piece of advice: "Is there anything else that you like besides Surgery? Because you should do that instead."

Then I thought for sure I would be a psychiatrist. I loved brains. Surgery was invasive, but Psychiatry was also invasive. Coming from a Psychology undergrad, analyzing people was second nature to me. The patients were interesting beyond belief, and I found plenty to write about, so I knew it would make an entertaining career. In particular, I felt at home with the idea of being a child psychiatrist—I had a knack for working with children, and I was inspired by their ability to heal and overcome. But I did not know just how difficult it would be. Halfway into my Child Psychiatry rotation, I was exhibiting symptoms of PTSD. I begrudgingly admitted that I did not have the mental resources to cope with the side effects of being a child psychiatrist.

Next on my list of "brainy specialties" was Neurology. I considered it only briefly. It wasn't part of the curriculum, so I didn't get a fair chance to explore it beyond my dealings with stroke and seizure patients. From what I gathered, the diagnostic aspect of Neurology was highly complex and elegant. But the treatment aspect was almost non-existent—for all the time spent figuring out exactly which part of the brain was damaged, there was usually nothing to be done about it.

From there, Pediatrics was a no-brainer (you guessed it—pun intended.) Cute sick kids, stuffed-animal stethoscope covers, doctors acting goofy in exchange for a peaceful listen to the heart and lungs. The idea of being happy all the time won me over almost instantly. Plus, this opened a new slew of possibilities for subspecialties: Pediatric Cardiology, Pediatric Endocrinology, Pediatric Whatever-ology. Since each of these would entail an additional three-year fellowship after residency, I was secretly buying myself more time to *really* decide what I wanted to be. (What? I like to dilly-dally over life-changing decisions!) It was a great plan, and I felt confident enough to start telling everybody about my decision. This was mid-January of my third year, and many of my classmates were jealous that I'd made up my mind so early. I went forward with it, collecting recommendation letters and setting up visiting internships, until August.

Because I kept telling myself that I loved children and hated adults, as pediatricians tend to do, I thought I was destined to hate my Internal Medicine rotation. As it turned out, I loved Internal Medicine because it was the first rotation in all of my medical training where I felt like I was personally and legitimately a doctor. Much of that feeling came from being introduced to the systematic approach to reading a chest X-ray.

We were taught by a pulmonologist whose hobbies happened to include Radiology and Physics. He opened his first lecture with a discussion of radiographic density. I believe "density" was the word that changed my destiny—it activated my inner Physics geek and thereby illuminated what had previously been a black box.

Radiology is glossed over in medical school. This is a mistake, because Radiology is ubiquitous and crucial to the practice of medicine—rarely is a diagnosis made without some kind of imaging. I may not have considered radiologists to be real doctors at the time, but I wasn't about to call myself a full-fledged doctor if I *didn't* have a proper understanding of Radiology. So I scheduled two full months of it right in the beginning of my fourth year.

Those two months were tumultuous. I started out with a lukewarm feeling: The work was engaging to varying degrees depending on who was teaching me, and sitting in a dark room all day was marginally tolerable. I often felt like I was watching other people play a video game that I didn't understand. That is, until one of the radiologists handed me a textbook to leaf through when times were slow. It was the best book I'd ever read in medical school, and I was raving about it to my husband when he asked for the millionth time if I was going into Radiology already. (My husband is himself a huge fan of Radiology.) I retorted that I did not come to medical school just to sit in an office and be nobody's doctor. But as I became more and more intrigued by what I was learning, I found myself in a dilemma. I started to question my commitment to Pediatrics, and indeed my whole paradigm of doctoring.

It was at this time that I re-read some of my old blog posts to start compiling this book, and I came across a piece I'd written about how to choose a specialty, called "How To Make Lifelong Decisions: Don't Compare Apples to Oranges. Just Make the Lemonade." (p. 116) I had forgotten all about this, and it took me completely by surprise. Apparently, I had figured out at some point that choosing a specialty wasn't about the nature of the work so much as about the kind of person I wanted to be—and I knew, undeniably, that radiologists were *exactly* the kind of people I wanted to emulate. Besides being the smartest of the smart, radiologists were sensible, sociable, happy, and generally wonderful to work with. And they all loved their families very much.

So then my gears were churning frantically. I only had a couple weeks left to submit my residency applications, and I had everything set up for Pediatrics. Radiology is a much more competitive specialty, and I frankly wasn't sure if I would be able to get in, especially with such little preparation. I finally came to the Dean of Student Affairs, Dr. Dupey, whom I consider the "Sorting Hat" of my medical school and to whom I give full credit for ensuring that we all match into residency.

She looked at my credentials and gave me the thumbs up! I still wasn't 100% ready to burn the bridge on Pediatrics, so she challenged me to write a personal statement for both (which I've included in the following pages.) I found it extremely easy to say why I wanted to go into Pediatrics; that essay took me about an hour. The Radiology one took me an entire weekend. I thought really hard, I got frustrated that my writing was inadequate to express my feelings, and I cried a lot. But when I emerged from this process, I was convinced that, one way or another, I would be a radiologist.

Seven grueling months later, I opened an envelope that fulfilled all my hopes and made all the trials worthwhile: I am going to Dartmouth to become a radiologist!

How to Make Lifelong Choices: Don't Compare Apples and Oranges. Just Make the Lemonade.

Every day, people ask me what I'm going to be when I grow up. For us kids in our mid-20's and 30's, this means which medical field we're going to specialize in when we graduate in a year and a half. To me this is a tough question, kind of like "What is the meaning of life?" The answer is a really big commitment.

But I've been going about it all wrong.

I thought that finding a specialty was like finding a husband: "In a perfect moment, I will simply *know* that my life was meant for _____." In my perfect specialty, I will maximize all of my talents, I will adore the patient population, I will save lives in the most glorious of ways, and I will be happy every single moment. I will withhold my decision until that specialty comes along. (Turns out, that's not how you find a husband either.)

It's not that those things won't be true in the life I choose. It's that those things don't come pre-packaged.

For me, and I think for most people, there are *many* ways to be happy. And this is why I've been running around in circles trying to figure out how to align my preferences: if I like cutting, if I like thinking, if I want to treat diabetes or gallbladders, etc., etc., etc. But that's like comparing apples and oranges when what you need to do is make some lemonade: It's not about your wish list. It's about making the best of what you're given. Because if you're opinionated enough, every last possible choice has at least one deal-breaker.

I've finally stopped thinking about what I want to do, and started thinking about the kind of person I want to be.

I want to be a good colleague. Someone who is kind, fun, and competent, who adapts easily to challenges, and who takes things in stride. I want to be a good wife and mother. One who listens and heals and strengthens. I can't afford to crash when I get home each day, or take out all my work anger on my family. I want to be a good person. I don't want to constantly yell at others to get their work done. I want to be the doctor who respects nurses, scrub techs, cafeteria workers... because we are all human beings. The answer then becomes obvious: I will choose something *less* stressful than what I think I can handle. Because whatever I do, I should do it with grace.

Truth is, I've seen enough frantic, stressed-out people who claim to be doing what they love most. Choosing a career is about finding a way to serve, uplift, and bring about the best in others. And these are *daily* choices, moment-to-moment choices. Obviously there is not a single specialty that would automatically make me all of the things I want to be. That's why it's dangerous to think that it's a once-in-a-lifetime choice: Once you've committed, the work has only just begun.

Pediatrics Personal Statement

I love working with children; I view it as my gift and my calling. Over the years, I have been engaged in various challenging and rewarding roles involving teaching and interacting with children: babysitting, volunteering in nurseries, teaching violin lessons, tutoring children with developmental disabilities, and, of course, "playing doctor" in my pediatric rotations. Children seem to like me instantly and respond readily when I teach concepts or give instructions. Ever since my earliest clinical experiences, I have known that I wanted to use this skill in my future career.

I entered medical school with an open mind, and have tried to explore as many medical specialties as I could schedule in the last three years. By immersing myself into each rotation as if it were going to be my life, I learned that I could come to love any specialty as long as I kept a good attitude. I learned that being happy every single day of my training was a decision rather than a set of circumstances. Though this initially complicated my process of choosing a specialty, I know that it will serve me well through the difficulties I will undoubtedly encounter in my career.

There are many specialties that I would find interesting, and I've been told repeatedly that being good with children does not necessitate a pediatric career. But ultimately I am choosing Pediatrics because that is where my heart is. Because I really believe in the worth of improving the lives of young patients, my interactions with children have been the most fulfilling aspect of any of my rotations. In particular, Pediatrics fits with my philosophy of what it means to be a doctor: to heal and affect positive change through personal relationships. During my summer preceptorship in Child Psychiatry, though I was saddened by the amount of damage that some of the patients had taken in their short lifespan, I found hope in their ability to form trusting relationships with their doctors who were able to guide them to move beyond their damage in a new, better direction. Children have a resilience, and potential for change and healing, unmatched by any other clinical population. I know that I have a greater potential to be a positive influence in someone's life as a pediatrician than in any other specialty.

Radiology Personal Statement

I am so happy to be choosing Radiology as the path to becoming the kind of doctor I've always envisioned: smart, cooperative, and compassionate.

I love that Radiology is "brainy," requiring great mental power and flexibility. Radiologists are central to the practice of medicine, as diagnoses and treatments so often pivot on the proper understanding of imaging. Of course, as a proper Physics geek, I am intrigued by the technology that continually increases our ability to know more and diagnose more. But what I love most about being on the cutting edge is the intellectual challenge of having familiar concepts swept out from under my feet. It's not enough to memorize the pathognomonic patterns—those may change along with advances in imaging modalities. For radiologists, there is a real advantage to reasoning by principles and not by rules; the difference being that a rule may forbid stepping off the roof, but the principle of gravity also extends to not jumping off a cliff.

I want to be a good colleague, one who uplifts and brings out the best in others. I've seen how a good radiologist can turn others into better doctors. During my Internal Medicine rotation, a very patient Radiology lecturer introduced me to the Physics principles of imaging and systematic approach to reading films, which opened my eyes to a new level of reasoning and sparked my interest in becoming a radiologist. In learning how shadows translate from densities, and densities from pathology, I finally began to illuminate what I previously saw as a mystery in medicine. I realized that there is an order and logic behind the shadows, revealing the answers to those who understand. I am excited not only to gain the diverse knowledge and skills that radiologists employ when consulted by physicians of all specialties, but also to continue working as part of a diverse team.

I want to be a good person, one who respects other people regardless of where they stand in the hierarchy. I love that Radiology, far from being an antisocial desk job, requires clinical skills and bedside manner. I was impressed that of all my mentors, it was a radiologist who stressed the importance of cleaning up my own sharps and treating nurses with respect, and who, in answer to a 90-year-old lady asking if he would recommend the thoracentesis, considered his own wife. Even though it may be easy to dehumanize the dozens of scans that populate the computer screen each day, I will not abandon my philosophy of what it means to be a doctor: to heal and affect positive change through personal relationships. I'm happy to know that a dark cubicle does not preclude this, but rather makes it even more important.

As I reviewed my experiences to choose my future, I realized that the answer lay much deeper than, "Do I like thinking or cutting? Do I want to treat diabetes or gallbladders?" What it took for me to love all my rotations was a good attitude, a strong work ethic, and a commitment to being happy. I know these qualities will serve me well in the difficulties that I will undoubtedly encounter in my career. Ultimately, my decision is based on the kind of person I want to be, and I look forward to residency as the next step in shaping that person. In this regard, I am seeking a program that will expand my boundaries, where I will grow intellectually, work as a productive member of a supportive team, and provide excellent patient care.

THE ADVENTURE CONTINUES

If you enjoyed reading this book, you can follow me to residency and beyond at www.uglydocling.com.

ABOUT THE AUTHOR

Marie Duan Meservy is a graduating University of Nevada medical student who writes about her diverse life adventures. Her story began in China where she was the child of two young doctors, living without refrigerators or hot water. She has since lived in Montreal and many parts of the U.S., and continues to broaden her perspective by traveling. She first decided to pursue medicine when, as an undergraduate, one of her research projects required her to perform open heart surgeries on mice. During her clinical years, she began writing stories about the brave and resilient patients she met in hospitals, but as her readers encouraged her to continually seek these lessons, this has blossomed into a passion that has shaped her practice of medicine. Her other passions include music, physics, baking, languages, teaching children, and helping others to choose happiness. This year, she has also taken on historical fencing, photography, and piano.